I0415804

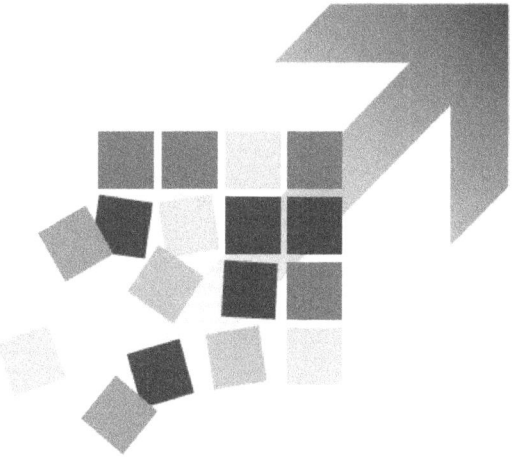

Proceedings from conference

From clinical trials to community:
The science of translating diabetes and obesity research

January 12-13, 2004

Natcher Conference Center
National Institutes of Health
Bethesda, Maryland

SPONSORS

National Institutes of Health

National Institute of Diabetes
and Digestive and Kidney Diseases

Office of Behavioral and
Social Sciences Research

**Centers for Disease
Control and Prevention**

Public Health Practice
Program Office

Division of Diabetes Translation

The sponsors of this conference would like to thank Dr. Roland G. Hiss of the Michigan Diabetes Research and Training Center for his insight, organizational and editing skills and Iain Mackenzie and Joe Vuthipong of the Hill Group for their hard work in making this report possible.

Annotated Table of Contents

Diabetes translation, and translation of any new biomedical or behavioral science, refers to the process through which new science is utilized to improve the nation's health. Translation occurs in two separate but sequential phases. Phase I Translation, usually dubbed "bench–to–bedside," applies basic scientific discoveries to human healthcare under controlled conditions, i.e., clinical research. Phase II Translation promotes the adoption of the fruits of promising clinical research by community-based healthcare under uncontrolled and (often) uncontrollable conditions.

Phase I Translation (bench–to–bedside) – usually defined as "clinical research" – are efficacy studies under controlled conditions with careful attention to internal validity. Phase II Translation (results of clinical research applied to community settings) are effectiveness trials in which promising clinical research is put to various reality tests in increasingly disparate settings, populations and circumstances. Translational research, as a special case of program evaluation and the ultimate effectiveness test, must take local circumstances into account while still striving for some generalizability.

Outcomes for translational research need to be practical, acceptable, and sensitive to intervention effects in addition to usual psychometric criteria such as internal consistency and reliability. Measures should include contextual factors, delivery of intervention components, hypothesized mediators, and both immediate and longer-term outcomes. A proposed generally applicable package of measurement categories for translational intervention evaluation should include: behavior change, quality of life, generalization (reach, adoption, and maintenance), implementation, economic outcomes and contextual factors.

Quality of life (QOL) is an important outcome for diabetes translational research. Several factors are associated with QOL for people with diabetes and they need to be taken into account as possible confounders or effect modifiers. There are several approaches to measuring QOL; each approach offers unique dimensions.

by rigorous qualitative and quantitative observational research. Nonrandomized study designs are frequently most appropriate for translational research, but all of these have methodologic trade-offs in terms of internal and external validity and bias. Given the complexity of changing systems of care, multi-factorial and multi-level interventions are needed to improve quality of care.

Economic evaluation is critical to controlling the cost and improving the efficiency of the healthcare system. Economic evaluation of medical care is most often approached using medical cost-effectiveness analysis. Several recent innovations in medical cost-effectiveness analysis – utility assessment, preference heterogeneity and self-selection, measurement of future cost, and use of value of information calculations to understand the potential value of research – all have potential relevance to cost-effectiveness in diabetes.

The research design should be closely linked to the purpose of the evaluation. Many promising designs for translational research build on a theoretical framework of behavioral change that is informed

Community-based participatory research (CBPR) brings together communities, researchers and agencies to improve health collaboratively in the community. All participants are equal partners, each bringing different strengths to the table. Sustaining efficacious diabetes care in real-world settings requires buy-in and individualization, which are features of CBPR efforts. CBPR may be especially useful for improving diabetes care in vulnerable, hard-to-reach populations.

Unless there is an explicit, formal model of how dissemination fits into the scientific process, it becomes a land to which no one travels. The highest level of a research organization must recognize and reinforce the importance of dissemination or translation. If we want to optimize likelihood of dissemination or translation, we should design for it. Usually, dissemination is an afterthought. Additionally, we must change the culture to make dissemination research a valued area of study and attention to dissemination an expected part of the research process.

Perspective of NIH Review Committees 42

Alan M. Delamater, PhD, *Professor of Pediatrics and Psychology, University of Miami School of Medicine*

The proposed intervention must address a significant public health issue and have a solid empirical basis in efficacy studies. The study approach should be directed to diverse populations; conducted in real-world settings; have an appropriate control group; use an intent-to-treat design; provide measures of implementation, including process measures such as treatment fidelity, staffing time and cost, and consumer and staff satisfaction; and include reliable, valid and clinically practical measures of both short and long-term outcomes, including health behaviors, health outcomes and quality of life. The investigators must have established a collaboration with the community-based organizations, have expertise with the proposed intervention, and have demonstrated the approach is feasible in the proposed setting.

Translational Research: The Medical Editor's View 45

Harold C. Sox, MD, MACP, *Editor, Annals of Internal Medicine*

Medical journals play an essential role in the evaluation and dissemination of clinical research. The process of scientific review and editing is labor intensive and costly. The article describes several issues concerning manuscript preparation, manuscript submission and manuscript review. The open access model of medical journalism provides free access to content and passes the cost of review from the subscriber to the author.

The model is unproven but currently under test. Publishing unbiased information about the effectiveness of new technology is an important public service. Achieving this goal requires constant attention.

Translating the Diabetes Prevention Program 49

David G. Marrero, PhD, *Professor of Medicine, Director, Diabetes Prevention and Control Center, Indiana University School of Medicine*

The Diabetes Prevention Program (DPP) demonstrated that type 2 diabetes can be delayed or possibly prevented by lifestyle modification and use of medication. The interventions, however, were not designed in a way that is directly deliverable on a public health scale. Translation on a public health scale will require: 1) increased community awareness of risk factors for diabetes and strategies for reducing them; 2) defining real-world strategies to identify individuals at risk who are likely to benefit most from lifestyle modifications; and 3) developing interventions or strategies to enhance dissemination and sustainability in nonresearch environments, particularly community venues where it can be accessed by broader segments of the population.

Translating Obesity and Diabetes Research: Some Challenges and Recommendations 53

Ken Resnicow, PhD, *Professor, School of Public Health, University of Michigan*

In the field of obesity, there is a disconnect between research interventions and clinical practice and formidable practitioner and system barriers to effective treatment exist. Recasting obesity as a behavioral rather than a medical condition is recommended to address these problems. This would involve switching the nexus of care to behavioral professionals. Redefining obesity as a cluster of heterogeneous conditions, termed "obesities", would foster a more individualized approach rather than the current one size fits all approach.

System change is necessary to translate science into clinical practice. Implementing, spreading and sustaining positive system change in health centers supports the need to address leadership, to transform clinical systems to a model of care and to apply strategies for learning and improvement. This systematic approach addresses formal, informal and technical aspects of care and organizational and personal behavior. Infrastructure and partnerships at the practice, state and national levels are essential to implement, support, sustain and spread positive change. Research methods need to address complex systems and not solely rely on understanding a system by splitting it into its component pieces.

Recent studies indicate that improvements in diabetes preventive behaviors ("intermediate process indicators") are occurring in most health systems, with early suggestions of stabilization of some long-term complications ("distal outcome indicators"). To continue improvements in the rate, depth and breadth of diabetes translation, however, 3 different realities must be addressed. *First*, changes must be made in existing health systems; *second*, serious commitment to prevention must occur; and *third*, continued excessive focus on individual entitlement to highly efficacious, expensive and specialty treatment (vs reasonable levels of broad-based communitarian health) will eventually undermine progress in diabetes translation.

The spectrum of scientific activities that begins with the identification of a health problem and ends with dissemination and translation of proven interventional approaches to the problem proceeds through 3 sequential steps: *Step 1* – epidemiologic and basic research to identify potential risk factors, mechanisms and influence; *Step 2* – clinical trials to determine efficacy of risk factor changes on health outcomes; *Step 3* – clinical and community trials to determine effectiveness of interventional approaches to change risk factors. The NIDDK has mounted a robust translational research program in support of each of these steps. The program includes: funding through the R18/R34 mechanism for translational research; Diabetes Research and Training Centers (DRTCs); Obesity and Nutritional Research Centers (ONRCs); Clinical Nutritional Research Centers (CNRUs); and participation in the recently established Obesity Research Task Force.

The fundamental need for an NIH "roadmap" to guide trans-NIH functions derives from the well-documented barriers moving scientific discovery from its origin (the "bench") to the bedside (clinical research) to the practice community nationwide (improvement of the nation's health). Efforts to establish the Roadmap began in August 2002 with consultation with over 100 thought leaders, followed by developmental discussions involving the NIH hierarchy and numerous outside collaborators, and leading to formal announcement of the Roadmap in September 2003. Three core themes characterize the NIH Roadmap: core theme #1, "New Pathways to Discovery"; core theme #2, "Research Teams of the Future"; and core theme #3, "Re-engineering Clinical Research".

Preface

This document was prepared to assist investigators in either academic or community-based organizations engaged in translational activities or translational research. In particular, this publication should be useful to applicants to either of the NIDDK announcements concerning translational research: "Translational Research for the Prevention and Control of Diabetes", PA-02-053 (R18 mechanism), and "Planning Grants for Translational Research for the Prevention and Control of Diabetes," PA-03-052 (R34 mechanism). All individuals interested in translational research funding opportunities should go to the NIDDK Web page for current initiatives and funding opportunities.

In September 2002, the Diabetes Mellitus Interagency Coordinating Committee (DMICC), congressionally charged with coordinating federal efforts in diabetes, conducted a one-day conference on the NIH Campus on the subject of diabetes translation. The DMICC conference examined several aspects of diabetes translation, a focus that underpins bringing the fruits of laboratory discoveries and clinical research to the patient and medical practice. A summary of this conference appears in *Diabetes Care* under the title "Considerations for Diabetes Translational Research in Real-World Settings" (*Diabetes Care* 26(9): 2670-2674, 2003).

The DMICC conference clarified the definition of diabetes translation, in particular noting that translation (of diabetes or other clinical science) occurs in two sequential phases: (1) application of basic laboratory-based research to clinical care, often called "bench-to-bedside" or "clinical research "; (2) widespread dissemination of the results of that clinical research to the community level with adoption of the new science by all individuals and populations (regardless of setting) who might benefit from it. The DMICC conference identified the need for a national conference to further explore the intricacies, challenges, barriers and rewards of research in this second phase of diabetes and obesity translation.

The national conference proposed by the DMICC was held January 12-13, 2004 on the NIH Campus and its proceedings are reported in this document. The conference examined challenges in complex situations facing providers caring for diverse communities with limited resources. Translation aims to determine what can improve outcomes in diverse, real-world populations and practically how to achieve those goals. Priority areas for diabetes and obesity translational research discussed at the conference included: the applicability of programs and results to different settings; understanding barriers and mediators to translation; how to move from an acute care paradigm to a chronic care model; vulnerable, understudied populations; translational interventions; community-based participatory research; economic analyses; and public health and public policy efforts.

It is clear that major societal benefits from basic and clinical research will not be realized unless translation of their findings to real-world practice occurs. Addressing diabetes translational issues effectively will require changes on the part of researchers, policy makers, funding organizations, grant review committees, and journal editorial boards.

Allen M. Spiegel, MD

Director
National Institute of Diabetes
and Digestive and Kidney Diseases
National Institutes of Health

Fundamental Issues in Translational Research

Translational Research – Two Phases of a Continuum

Roland G. Hiss, MD

Professor Emeritus of Medical Education
(formerly, Coordinator of Prevention and

*Control Division of the Michigan Diabetes
Research and Training Center)
University of Michigan Medical School*

Key Points

1. Diabetes translation, and translation of any new biomedical or behavioral science, refers to the process through which that new science is utilized to improve the nation's health. Translation occurs in two separate but sequential phases.

2. *Phase One Translation*, usually dubbed "bench-to-bedside," applies basic scientific discoveries to human health care under controlled conditions, i.e. clinical research.

3. *Phase Two Translation* promotes the adoption of the fruits of promising clinical research by community–based health care under uncontrolled and (often) uncontrollable conditions.

4. Section One of this document, Fundamental Issues in Translational Research, addresses multiple issues associated with the selection, design, planning, conduct and outcome measurement of *Phase Two Translational Research*.

The Translation Movement of the Last Quarter Century

The Diabetes Mellitus Research in Education Act of 1974 (PL-93-354), hereinafter "the act", initiated a comprehensive, national diabetes program that has guided the Federal Government's approach to diabetes over the last quarter century. The central element of the act provided for a National Commission on Diabetes to "formulate a long-range plan to combat diabetes mellitus with specific recommendations for the utilization and organization of national resources for that purpose." The act also amended the Public Health Service Act in several significant ways, specifically:

1. Provision of diabetes mellitus prevention and control programs (later implemented by the Centers for Disease Control and Prevention);

2. Development or expansion of centers of research and training in diabetes mellitus and related endocrine and metabolic disorders (later Diabetes Research and Training Centers [DRTCs], and Diabetes Endocrinology Research Centers [DERCs]); and

3. Recommendations for a "diabetes coordinating committee" (later the Diabetes Mellitus Interagency Coordinating Committee, or DMICC).

The Commission, chaired by Oscar B. Crofford, MD, met throughout calendar 1975. Across the nation, the Commission gathered testimony from the diabetes community – healthcare professionals, diabetes researchers both basic and clinical, healthcare delivery systems large and small, and, most importantly, hundreds of persons with diabetes and their families.

The landmark report of the National Commission on Diabetes, dated December 1975, provided Congress with a comprehensive blueprint – the "long-range plan" – for Federal initiatives in

diabetes for the last quarter of the 20th century. The Commission fleshed out key provisions of the 1974 Act, notably: 1) that the National Institute of Health establish diabetes research and training centers (DRTCs); 2) that the Centers for Disease Control (and Prevention) support diabetes control programs within state public health departments; 3) that the Diabetes Mellitus Interagency Coordinating Committee (DMICC) be formed to coordinate the diabetes-related activities of multiple Federal agencies. In addition, the Commission recommended that the NIH undertake a concerted effort to determine the consequences of sustained hyperglycemia (later conducted as the Diabetes Control and Complications Trial, DCCT), and that the NIH and the private sector provide increased funding for basic and clinical research in diabetes.

A principal charge to diabetes research and training centers, as articulated by the National Commission, was to: *translate the advances in the field of diabetes research with least delay into improved care for the diabetic (sic) in the setting of model care demonstration within the centers* (now called Phase One translation) *and through outreach programs in the regional community* (now called Phase Two translation)."

The term "translate" had its origin in the 1975 National Commission on Diabetes report. The struggle to define "translate," or "translation" in the noun form, and to understand the far-reaching concepts these words embrace has both inspired and confused the diabetes community (and that of many other behavioral and bio-medical disciplines) in the nearly three decades since they were introduced. The diabetes translational research conference *From Clinical Trials to Community: The Science of Translating Diabetes and Obesity Research* held on the NIH campus in January 2004 – the proceedings of which are set forth in this document – explored current understanding of the concept of diabetes translation and stimulated creative thought on how and why further research in this important area might be pursued.

Translation Is a Two-Phase Process

Diabetes translation, and translation of any new biomedical or behavioral science, refers to the process through which that new science is utilized to improve the nation's health. Translation occurs in two separate but sequential phases, as defined in Key Points number 2 and 3 above. Phase One Translation receives enormous attention and research funding and is conducted in a rigorous and controlled fashion (as it should be). Phase Two Translation, in contrast, has received little attention (except for naïve expressions of intent), little research funding, and is extremely difficult to do in a controlled fashion. Until recently, Phase Two Translation was not even recognized as part of the translational process and was not included in its definition. From a societal perspective, the imbalance of research efforts between Phase One and Phase Two Translation carries enormous cost, as the true measure of the social value of brilliant new biomedical and behavioral science relates to improvement of the nation's health, not just the acquisition and archiving of new knowledge.

Naturally Occurring Phase Two Translation Is Chaos

A reasonable observer might assume that promising new biomedical and behavioral science would be quickly and universally offered to any patient who might benefit from it. The power of the new science to improve the human condition should be sufficient, the reasonable observer assumes, to propel widespread adoption of the new science by those providing health care and the patients they serve. Unfortunately, this is rarely the case. In the real world, Phase Two Translation stumbles unguided towards a very uneven, extraordinarily incomplete, and socially disappointing state of affairs.

Awareness Is Not Adoption

There is a common belief that Phase Two Translation is a matter of information dissemination. If we "get the word out," widespread adoption of "the word" will occur. This belief drives multitudinous, well-intentioned information dissemination activities: the medical literature; national, regional and local clinical scientific meetings in all kinds of formats; the CME industry; the Internet; educational programs of every conceivable type, from simple fact sheet or brochure to large national, interactive, computerized programs; and many others. All of these information dissemination activities are useful and a reasonable first step in Phase Two Translation. However, they are far from sufficient to accomplish adoption of new science into everyday practice. They merely produce a vague awareness that the new science exists and even their performance in that regard is marginal in terms of target audience reached. The many target audiences of information dissemination efforts regard them as intellectual spam. They were not requested and they don't address "my problems." *Information dissemination does not address the conditions and circumstances of the target audiences involved and therefore does little to convert awareness into adoption.*

It's Not My Job

Phase One Translation has a thousand mothers and fathers. Phase Two Translation is an orphan. Biomedical and behavioral research scientists, and the institutions that support them, believe that scientific discovery and its proper archiving constitutes the totality of their responsibilities. There is no doubt they take these responsibilities very seriously and execute them magnificently. But who/what takes the next step? At this point, very few. Congress and the American people ask why.

A Final Quibble About Words . . .

Translation – *a noun*, encompasses the myriad of steps necessary to ensure that the full social value of the biomedical and behavioral science is realized through improvement in the nation's health.

Translate – *a verb*, performing the acts of translation.

Translational – *an adjective*, qualifying a noun (such as research, intervention, analysis, discussion, etc.) as dealing with translation.

This document concerns *translational research* in diabetes and obesity.

References

Garfield SA, Malozowski S, Chin MH, Venkat Narayan KM, Glasgow RE, Green LW, Hiss RG, Krumholz HM. Considerations for diabetes translational research in real-world settings. *Diabetes Care* 26(9): 2670-2674, 2003.

Hiss RG. The concept of diabetes translation: Addressing barriers to widespread adoption of new science into clinical care. *Diabetes Care* 24(7): 1293-1296, 2001.

Lenfant C. Clinical research to clinical practice – Lost in translation? *NEJM* 349(9): 868-874, 2003.

Sung NG, Crowley WF, Genel M et al. Central challenges facing the national clinical research enterprise. *JAMA* 289(10): 1278-1287, 2003.

From Efficacy to Effectiveness to Community and Back: Evidence-Based Practice vs Practice-Based Evidence

Lawrence W. Green, DrPH

Director, Office of Science and Extramural Research
Public Health Practice Program Office
Centers for Disease Control and Prevention

Judith M. Ottoson, EdD, MPH

Associate Professor
Andrew Young School of Policy Studies
Georgia State University

Key Points

1. In the cycle of research to practice and back, several types of evidence accumulate from efficacy trials and are put to various reality tests in increasingly disparate settings, populations, and circumstances.

2. As evidence from highly controlled efficacy trials (Phase One Translation), in the robes of "best practice," confronts various realities of community-based practice and uncontrolled circumstances, it must be translated and put to tests other than internal validity.

3. Research concerning Phase Two Translation, as a special case of program evaluation and the ultimate effectiveness test, must take local circumstances into account while still striving for some generalizability.

4. The art and science of Phase Two Translation must balance respect for the scientific rigor of previous research (Phase One Translation) with respect for indigenous wisdom about the local situation. More community participatory approaches to this phase of translational research help achieve this balance.

Efficacy vs Effectiveness

Much of the confusion about the differences in purpose and methods of the two sequential phases of the translational process relates to confusion about the differences in purpose and methods of *efficacy vs effectiveness* studies. The following definitions may clarify this confusion.

Efficacy: The tested impact of an intervention under highly controlled circumstances. Efficacy studies maximize internal validity, i.e., the degree to which one can conclude with confidence that the intervention caused the result. Clinical efficacy studies are often dubbed "bench-to-bedside," more appropriately designated "clinical research." Clinical research is Phase One of the translational process that attempts to bring new science (from whatever source) to clinical application under controlled circumstances and using rigorous scientific methods.

Effectiveness: The tested impact of an intervention under real-world circumstances (relatively uncontrolled, real-time, "typical" settings, populations and conditions). Effectiveness studies maximize external validity, i.e., the degree to which one can generalize from the test to other times, places, or populations. The methods employed in effectiveness studies may have the appearance of being "less rigorous," at least to the traditionally schooled investigative scientist and his/her peer reviewers.

The Cycle of Research to Practice and Back

Research typically proceeds towards practice from the sincere attempts to disseminate findings from highly controlled trials. The failure of much of the accumulated research to penetrate community-based practice cycles back to the research enterprise as a demand for more technologically sophisticated and affordable efficient solutions that impose less of a burden on practitioners, payers, patients, consumers, or the at-risk public. Some of the frustrations of practitioners cycle in a short-loop feedback to health program managers and policy makers as a plea for more help in translating research to the realities of practice, financing the necessary supports for evidence-based practices, and reorganizing the conditions of practice to accommodate them.

Traditional Randomized Controlled Trials (RCTs) in Phase Two Translational Research

The randomized control trial (RCT) performs exceedingly well as the gold standard for research methodology in Phase One Translation (efficacy studies, controlled clinical research). However, the utility of the RCT in Phase Two Translational research (effectiveness studies under less controlled real-world conditions) has been challenged on a number of grounds. A review of the strengths of an RCT in controlled clinical research and the caveats on its application to uncontrolled real-world research is in order.

Strengths of an RCT

1. Utilizes a sample of the target population or intended recipients of the intervention (the application of the new science to the human condition).

2. Randomly assigns the sample population to experimental and control groups, the former to receive the intervention, the latter to be unexposed to it.

3. Employs appropriate pre and post intervention measures to assess effect of the intervention in the experimental group not seen in the control group.

4. When employed in clinical research, can be used to formulate "best practices" as a guide to generation of effectiveness studies in real-world conditions.

Caveats to Employing RCT Methods in Real-World Settings

1. Problems applying (translating) "best practices" to real-world community of practitioners, health care agencies and patients – all of whom ask: a) Do I have the same resources as the experimenters? (Usually no.) b) How different is the experimenter's situation from mine? (Usually quite.) c) Is it really necessary and realistic for me to strive for such lofty goals in my practice (or life)? (Philosophical question.)

2. Problems inherent in generalizing from research in one place, with one population, to other places and circumstances.

3. Problems associated with applying "best practices" to underserved populations and the less educated, less affluent – and possibly differently motivated than the original participants of the efficacy study that generated the "best practices."

Breaking the Logjam Separating Efficacy Trials (Research Center) from Effectiveness Trials (Community)

The factors (barriers) that clog the pipeline from research center-based clinical research to community-based practice are numerous: a) the types of research products flowing from efficacy trials; b) bias toward internal validity in the effectiveness trials; c) oversimplification of the causal mechanisms at work in social and behavioral systems; d) poor fit at the community-based practice end of the original efficacy trial research product.

A successful bridge from efficacy to effective trials (Phase Two Translation) must address all of these "logjams." The approach to creating this "successful bridge" requires a very different paradigm than the traditional RCT. The "laboratory" in this paradigm is the community and the "research subjects" are the highly varied, free-living inhabitants of that community. Effectiveness studies conducted in that laboratory with these subjects require considerable planning, team building, pre intervention assessments, and most particularly:

1. Determination of the joint overlap of three factors – the population's perceived needs and priorities, their actual needs, and the available resources to effect change. Only interventions that address all three of these factors are feasible in community-based research;

2. Development of a highly functional research center/community partnership, called a coalition;

3. Development of a coalition-led research plan that emphasizes:

a) control by practitioners, patient, client, community or population;
b) local evaluation and monitoring;
c) systematic study of place, setting and culture; and
d) regards "best practice" as a process rather than a packaged intervention: the diagnostic-planning-evaluation cycle.

A fairly recently defined term for the paradigm of community-based effectiveness trials is *participatory research*, described in the next section.

Participatory Research as Translational Research (or vice versa)

Part of the solution to the research relevance issues in closing the gap between research and practice surely lies in closer consultation, if not in engagement, of practitioners or other end users in the research enterprise. Participatory research has enjoyed various incarnations in government-sponsored and foundation-sponsored initiatives in community development, health promotion programs, and most recently in collaborative clinical trials in family practice and pediatrics. This approach to effectiveness studies in community-based translational efforts can serve the purpose of getting a better fit between science and practice.

A later chapter in this document entitled "Community-Based Participatory Research for Diabetes Translation and Multi-level, Multi-factorial Interventions" authored by Marshall Chin expands on the principles, methods, and experience with the participatory research approach.

References

Cameron R et al. Linking science and practice: Toward a system for enabling communities to adopt best practices for chronic disease prevention. *Health Prom Practice*, 2001; 2:35-42.

Glasgow R et al. Why don't we see more translation of health promotion research to practice? Rethinking the efficacy-to-effectiveness transition. *Am J Public Health*, 2003; Aug; 93(8), 1261-7.

Green LW. From research to "best practices" in other settings and populations (American Academy of Health Behavior Research Laureate address). *American Journal of Health Behavior*, 2001; 25, 165-78. Full text online at *http://www.ajhb.org/2001/number3/25-3-2.htm*

Green LW, Kreuter MW. *Health Program Planning: An Educational and Ecological Approach*, 4th Ed. New York: McGraw Hill Higher Education, 2005.

Green LW, Mercer SM. Can public health researchers and agencies reconcile the push from funding bodies and the pull from communities? *Am J Public Health*, 2001 Dec; 91: 1926-9.

Minkler M et al. Community-based participatory research: Implications for public health funding. *Am J Public Health*, 2003 Aug; 93: 1210-3.

Ottoson JM. (1997) Beyond transfer of training: Using multiple lenses to assess community education programs. In Rose, A.D. & M.A. Leahy (eds.). New Directions for Adult and Continuing Education 75, 87-96.

Ottoson JM. Reclaiming the concept of application: From social to technological process and back again. *Adult Education Quarterly*, 1995; 46, 1-30.

Section II
Outcomes for Translational Research

What Outcomes Are Most Important for Translational Research?

Russell E. Glasgow, PhD

Senior Scientist
Kaiser Permanente Colorado

Key Points

1. Measures for translational research need to be practical, acceptable, and sensitive to intervention effects in addition to usual psychometric criteria such as internal consistency and reliability.

2. Constructing a logic model of an intervention and its intended effects will often be helpful in identifying measures and should include contextual factors, intervention components, hypothesized mediators, and both immediate and longer term outcomes.

3. Translational research issues are complex and multi-faceted. Often an intervention that does well on one criterion may do poorly on others. Thus, a package of measures is recommended rather than a single primary outcome measure.

4. A proposed generally applicable package of measurement categories for translational intervention evaluation should include measures of: behavior change, quality of life, generalization (reach, adoption, and maintenance), implementation, economic outcomes, and contextual factors.

Need for Practical, Sensitive Measures

Measurement schemes for translational research need to recognize the differences between efficacy and effectiveness research, and also the importance of partnerships among researchers, participants, and setting administrators, clinicians and decision makers. This usually means that there are major time, modality, and cost limitations as well as acceptability issues to consider. Many of the 'state of the art' measures are too time consuming, intrusive or expensive to use in large scale translational and community-based studies. Another issue is that in interventional studies, the primary concern is whether an intervention produces significant improvement compared to a control condition. Thus, it is critical that the measures used be sensitive to change. This is a different emphasis than in much basic research in which the emphasis is primarily on criteria such as internal consistency. Some measures may have strong traditional psychometric characteristics, but be insensitive to change or intervention effects.

Logic Models Can Be Useful

The Guide to Community Preventive Services coordinated by the Centers for Disease Control and Prevention (CDC) uses a 'logic model' to diagram and understand likely effects of an intervention when planning literature reviews. Such a model can also help in deciding upon the most important measures to include in a translational research study. A logic model specifies the sequential effects that can be expected due to contextual and moderating factors, interventional components, mediating variables (the path or process through which an intervention is hypothesized to achieve its impact), and both short and longer term outcomes. Logic models can be used to inform selection of measures and to identify specific steps or links in the hypothesized sequence for which there are or are not supporting data.

Translational Outcomes Are Complex and Multifaceted

As illustrated in the RE-AIM framework (Reach, Effectiveness, Adoption, Implementation, and Maintenance) there are multiple factors that contribute to the ultimate impact and public health or population-based effects of an intervention. (A full description for the RE-AIM framework [*http://www.re-aim.org*] and its contribution to planning and evaluating phase two translational research may be found in Glasgow et al, 2001.)

In translational research, attention needs to be extended beyond just efficacy (effects on a single dependent variable) to multiple outcomes. Among the reasons for this are that outcome measures for diabetes are not highly correlated; interventional programs that do well on one dimension may actually do worse on other important criteria. Furthermore, different stakeholders and decision makers are often interested in different outcomes (e.g., clinical outcomes vs. cost; patient-centered outcomes vs. organizational outcomes; short-term vs. long-term). In translational research intended to have real world implications, there is seldom a single best outcome measure – rather it is necessary to evaluate results from multiple perspectives and across a variety of measures.

Outcome/Measurement Issues To Consider When Planning Phase Two Translational Research

(Adopted form Tunis, Stryer and Clancy, *JAMA* 2003)

1. In practical clinical trials, the study sample should be diverse (*reach*).

• Few exclusion criteria.
• Representative on racial, ethnic, age, gender, and other sociodemographic factors.
• Representative of typical and complex patients.
• Includes those in primary care having comorbidities, taking medications, having depression.

2. The study should take place in multiple representative settings (*adoption*).

• Multiple community settings.
• Includes typical nonresearch community-based staff.
• Relevant to primary care.
• Report variations in process and outcomes across settings.

3. The study should address multiple health outcomes.

• More than knowledge and A1c.
• Outcomes relevant to patients, purchasers, clinicians, policy makers, and the public.
• Quality of life.
• Economic outcomes.

4. There are measurement obligations not usually encountered in phase one translational (clinical) research.

• Time Spent – each step and overall.
• Expense – direct, indirect and diverted (using up of care provider and patient time and attention).
• Intervention delivery (*implementation*) by staff with different levels of training and expertise.

A Proposed Measurement Package for Translational Research

Considering the above perspectives and the information needed by policy-makers prior to widespread adoption of a "best practice" or other quality improvement intervention, six categories of measurement are proposed for inclusion in most translational intervention research. Two of these categories – 1) contextual factors (often qualitative and interpretive) and 2) implementation – do not produce any burden on patient participants. Two other measurement categories – 3) generalization (reach, adoption, maintenance) and 4) economic measures – can be estimated using records if planned for prior to the study. The final two measures – 5) behavior change (of patients and clinical staff) and 6) quality of life – are central to the purpose of translational research and are the subject of much current research to identify optimal measures. The specific measure(s) within each category should be tailored to the purpose and content of each particular study, though there is value for the field if common measures are used across studies.

In summary, there are no easy answers to the question "what are the best measures to use in my translational research study?", but the above criteria provide a useful framework and set of guidelines for selecting measures. The real world is complex, contextual and multi dimensional. If our measures are to be relevant to this challenge, they should also have these characteristics.

References

Centers for Disease Control and Prevention (2004). *The Guide to Community Preventive Services. http://www.thecommunityguide.org* (Accessed July 20, 2004).

Farquhar CM, Stryer D, Slutsky J. Translating research into practice: The future ahead. *International Journal for Quality Health Care*, 2002; 14, 223-249.

Glasgow RE. Translating research to practice: Lessons learned, areas for improvement, and future directions. *Diabetes Care*, 2003; 26: 2451-6.

Glasgow RE, Lichtenstein E, Marcus AC. Why don't we see more translation of health promotion research to practice? Rethinking the efficacy to effectiveness transition. *American Journal of Public Health*, 2003; 93: 1261-1267.

Glasgow RE, McKay HG, Piette JD, Reynolds KD. The RE-AIM framework for evaluating interventions: What can it tell us about approaches to chronic illness management? *Patient Education and Counseling*, 2001; 44, 119-127.

Green LW. An interview with Lawrence W. Green [interview by Molly T. Laflin and David R. Black]. *Am J Health Behav*. 2003 Jul-Aug; 27(4):466-78.

Tunis SR, Stryer DB, Clancey CM. (2003). Practical clinical trials: Increasing the value of clinical research for decision making in clinical and health policy. *JAMA*, 290, 1624-1632.

Quality of Life Outcomes in Translation

K. M. Venkat Narayan, MD, MPH, MBA

Division of Diabetes Translation
Centers for Disease Control and Prevention

Key Points

1. Quality of life (QOL) is an important outcome for diabetes translational research.

2. Several factors are associated with QOL in people with diabetes and they need to be taken into account as possible confounders or effect modifiers.

3. There are several approaches to measuring QOL; each approach offers unique dimensions.

Importance of QOL

Several factors make QOL an important outcome for chronic diseases such as diabetes. The increasing prevalence of chronic diseases in our society is shifting emphasis from objective measures of health (mortality and morbidity) to subjective measures (Health-Related Quality of Life, SRH). The perspective of the patient is gaining importance, first with greater respect for patient autonomy and right to choose among medical options (1940s-1980s), to focus on patient-centered outcomes and patient-defined goals of medical care (1980s-2000s). In addition, the growth in the importance of economics and changes in the organization and delivery of health care also make QOL an important outcome.

Several Factors Affect QOL in People with Diabetes

People with diabetes have worse quality of life than those without, but better QOL than people with other serious chronic illnesses. Among people with diabetes, QOL is not associated with duration or type; not impaired by intensive treatment; strongly impaired by complications; associated with some demographic factors (e.g., age, gender, education); and associated with health status and perceived ability to control diabetes.

Approaches to Measuring QOL

QOL is a multi-dimensional construct. Measures of QOL fall into two categories: illness-specific and global. The illness-specific measures focus on problems specific to diabetes (e.g., hypoglycemia, insulin injections). Several diabetes-specific measures are available (e.g., Diabetes quality of life, DQOL; Diabetes-39; Problem areas in diabetes, PAID; Diabetes treatment satisfaction questionnaire, DTSQ).

The global measures are useful for making comparisons across health and illness groups. The concepts related to global measures are health-related quality of life (HRQOL), quality-adjusted life years (QALY), and willingness-to-pay.

From clinical trials to community:
The science of translating diabetes and obesity research

Specific Measures of Global QOL

1. Health Related Quality of Life (HRQOL)

HRQOL refers to the impact of health aspects of an individual's life on that person's quality of life, or overall wellbeing, or refers to the value of a health state to an individual. There are two ways of measuring HRQOL: a) non-preference-based approach (called a "health profile"), and b) preference-based approach (called a "utility measure").

Nonpreference-based HRQOL instruments measure physical, social and role functioning that capture behavioral dysfunction; they also measure mental states, perceptions of overall health, and pain that reflect subjective components. Nonpreference-based HRQOL instruments cannot produce a single (composite) score nor can they be used for economic evaluations. Examples include the Medical Outcomes Study General Health Survey Short-Forms (SF-36, SF-20 and SF-12).

Preference-based HRQOL employ an elicitation method that is rooted in the axioms of expected utility theory. An individual (or a community or a health professional) is asked to choose between a less desirable (but certain) chronic health state and a "gamble" offering a certain probability of a worse health state (dead) or having an improved state of health (healthy). A preference-based HRQOL may also employ a time trade-off approach to determine how many years of life in excellent health are equivalent to life in a less desirable state. Examples of preference-based HRQOL instruments

include: Quality of well being, QWB; Health utility index, HUI; and European quality of life scale, EUROQOL.

2. Quality-Adjusted Life Years (QALY)

A QALY is a summary outcome measure that incorporates the quality or utility of a health state with the duration of survival. A QALY combines two possible effects of a disease or an intervention – extending life or improving the health-related quality of life – in a multiplicative way.

To calculate a QALY, the researcher assigns a number that corresponds to the quality of health state during each period during the survival, where 1.0 represents optimal health and 0 is dead. The scores (utilities) are then added across time periods.

The following scheme demonstrates how QALY calculation shows benefit of a hypothetical intervention.

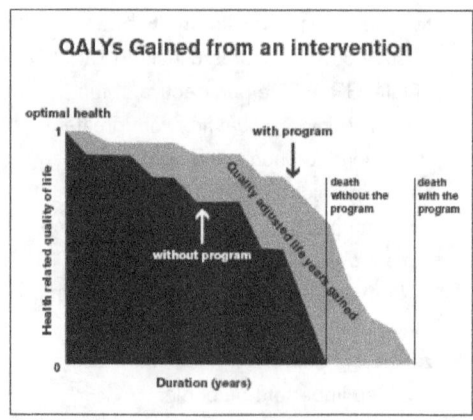

QALYs Gained from an intervention

optimal health

Health related quality of life

with program

death without the program

death with the program

without program

Duration (years)

3. Willingness-to-Pay for Health Benefits (WTP)

The WTP method of calculating global HRQOL measures the value an individual places on reducing risk of death or illness by estimating the maximum dollar amount an individual would pay in a given risk-reduction situation. Using survey methods, respondents are presented with hypothetical scenarios about a health benefit and asked to imagine that an actual market exists for the benefit and then state the maximum they would be willing to pay for it under various contingency conditions.

As an example, assume you are an infertile female and want to have a baby and are told that in vitro fertilization can help if purchased. You express a WTP of $17,000 (if 10% chance of success is offered), $28,000 (if 25% chance of success) and $43,000 (if 50% chance). This results in an implied WTP of $177, 000 per statistical baby.

References

Haddix AC. Prevention effectiveness: A guide to decision analysis and economic evaluation. Oxford University Press, NY, 1996.

Neumann PJ, Johannesson M The willingness to pay for in vitro fertilization: A pilot study using contingent valuation. *Med Care* 1994 Jul;32(7):686-99.

Rubin RR, Peyrot M. Quality of life and diabetes. *Diabetes/Metabolism Research and Reviews* 1999;15:205-218.

Methodological Issues in Economic Evaluation

David Meltzer, MD, PhD

Associate Professor
Department of Medicine, School of Public

Policy and Department of Economics.
Director, MD/PhD Program in the Social
Sciences and RWJ Clinical Scholars Program
University of Chicago

Key Points

1. Economic evaluation is critical to controlling the cost and improving the efficiency of the health care system.

2. Economic evaluation of medical care is most often approached using medical cost-effectiveness analysis, which has theoretical foundations in microeconomic theory.

3. Several recent innovations in medical cost-effectiveness analysis – relating to utility assessment, preference heterogeneity and self-selection, the measurement of future costs, and the use of value of information calculations to understand the potential value of research – all have potential relevance to cost-effectiveness in diabetes.

Background

In the past 40 years, there have been enormous increases in health care costs. In nominal terms, these costs have risen from $28 billion in 1960 to $1.5 trillion today (2004). As a percentage of gross national product (GNP), this represents a rise from 5% to 14%. During these 40 years, health care spending has grown by 2.5% more per year than the rest of the economy.

The reasons for these increases in health care costs fall into two categories: 1) growth in quantity of health care provided nationally

(1.6% per year), and 2) growth in prices charged (0.9% per year). Much of the growth in prices is related to growth in quantity as quality-adjusted prices are actually falling. Growth in health care costs has stimulated demand for cost-effectiveness analysis from several quarters: academic medicine; government (especially foreign governments); private payers; and pharmaceutical companies (who refer work in this area as "pharmacoeconomics").

Rationale for Economic Evaluation

There is strong evidence that the use of medical technology is the primary driver of increasing the costs and that the incremental value of those new technologies is variable. Economic evaluation can provide data to inform efficient allocation of resources and control costs in any health care setting by providing a systematic approach to assess the benefits of specific health interventions relative to their costs.

Role of Medical Cost-Effectiveness Analysis in Economic Evaluation

Medical cost-effectiveness analysis is the most commonly used approach for economic evaluation in health care. The most common theoretical framework for medical cost-effectiveness analysis uses quality-adjusted life years to measure health benefits, reflecting effects on both the length and quality of life. Although there are a series of theoretical and empirical questions about the value of this framework, it is by far the most widely used approach of its kind and has been applied in an incredibly wide range of medical interventions.

Several methodologic issues arise in cost-effectiveness analyses (CEA) as described below.

1. Type of Analysis:

a) Cost minimization: the least expensive method to accomplish a fixed objective, which depends on the problematic assumption that the objective should be met.

b) Cost-benefit: measurement of costs and benefits in dollar terms selecting all treatments for which the net benefit is greater than zero. This method places a dollar value on outcomes, which may be controversial in some applications.

c) Cost-effectiveness: compares the change in cost to the change in benefit (Δ costs/Δ benefits) and permits selection of treatment options for a given situation to those with the lowest cost effectiveness ratios. CEA is useful in situations where both costs and effectiveness are decreasing *or* both costs and effectiveness are increasing. (It is self-apparent that when costs increase and effectiveness decreases the treatment should *never* be performed; conversely, when costs decrease and effectiveness increases, the treatment is *always* advisable.)

2. Perspective – Methodological issues involved in cost-effective analyses vary considerably depending upon the perspective of the agency conducting the analysis. These perspectives can be categorized into private (e.g. health care providers and consumers), public (e.g. Medicare, Medicaid, state mental health systems) and societal in which all costs and benefits are included no matter to whom they accrue.

3. Definition and Measurement of Benefits – Benefits may be determined for specific outcomes, e.g. cancers detected or cancers cured, or general outcomes. The most common method for measuring benefits of general outcomes is Quality-Adjusted Life Years (QALYs) saved in which a "life year" is weighted by quality of life weights between 0 (death) and 1 (perfect health).

As noted above, although many theoretical and empirical questions about the contribution of QALYs to cost-effectiveness analysis remain unresolved, they presently are the gold standard for benefit measurement and have been used in more than 1,000 medically diverse studies.

Importance of Methodological Innovations in Medical Cost-Effectiveness Analysis

Several important methodological issues in medical cost-effectiveness analysis that have been areas of recent research have important implications for the economic evaluation of treatments for diabetes.

1. Utility Assessment – Utility measures are often based on psychometric techniques that may or may not have much empirical content. An alternative approach is to consider patient choices as a revelation of their preferences. Although this approach also has concerns associated with it, in the case of diabetes, it

has provided some evidence that the burden associated with current therapies may have been under-appreciated in some economic analyses of treatments for diabetes.

2. Preference Heterogeneity and Self-Selection – If patient preferences are used in economic evaluation, variation in those preferences is inevitable. Sensitivity analysis is sometimes used, but it is not always clear how to interpret such results when cost-effectiveness is preference sensitive. A related issue is that people (patients in this case) may systematically self-select treatments based on their preferences, causing interventions to be more cost-effective in practice than suggested by standard decision models. New evidence suggests that such self-selection has dramatic effects on the cost-effectiveness of intensive therapy among the elderly, changing it from harmful on average in some analysis to beneficial and highly cost-effective.

3. Future Costs – There has been a long-standing controversy about whether to include future medical costs for unrelated illnesses and future non-medical costs in medical cost-effectiveness analyses. Recent theoretical advances have shown that such costs should be included and that failing to do so often biases analyses to favor interventions that extend life over interventions that improve quality of life, especially among interventions that extend life at older ages. Interventions in diabetes are influenced in this framework in complex ways because of potential effects on length of life versus quality of life and because affected individuals may be of all ages, altering the magnitude and direction of future medical costs.

4. Value of Research – Medical decision analysts and health economists have recently been increasingly interested in understanding the value of biomedical research. Several complementary methods have been used to try to understand the value of improved health overall and to provide data to inform decisions about research priorities. None of this research to date has focused on diabetes but it appears to be an obvious area for future work.

References

Meltzer D. Accounting for future costs in medical cost-effectiveness analysis. *Journal of Health Economics* 16 (1): 33-64, 1997.

Meltzer D. Addressing uncertainty in medical cost-effectiveness analysis: Implications of expected utility maximization for methods to perform sensitivity analysis and the use of cost-effectiveness analysis to set priorities for medical research. *Journal of Health Economics* 20(1):109-129, 2001.

Meltzer D, Polonsky T. Do quality-adjusted life years reflect patient preferences? Validation using revealed preference for intensive treatment of insulin-dependent diabetes mellitus. *Medical Decision Making* 18: 459, October 1998.

Meltzer D, Huang E, Jin L, Shook M, Chin M. Major bias in cost-effectiveness analysis due to failure to account for self-selection: Impact in intensive therapy for type 2 diabetes among the elderly. *Med Decis Making.* 2003; 23(6): 576.

Section III
Experimental Design Issues in Translational Research

Linkage of Question to Design for Diabetes Translation

Carol M. Mangione, MD, MSPH

Professor of Medicine; Director,
Resource Center for Minority Aging Research
David Geffen School of Medicine at UCLA

Key Points

1. The research design should be closely linked to the purpose of the evaluation.

2. Many of the most promising designs for translational research build on a theoretical framework of behavioral change that is informed by rigorous qualitative and quantitative observational research.

3. Nonrandomized study designs or randomized designs that are above the level of the participant are frequently most appropriate for translational research but all of these have methodological trade-offs in terms of internal and external validity and bias.

4. Given the complexity of changing systems of care, multi-factorial and multi-level interventions are needed to improve quality of care.

Linkage of the Research Design to the Purpose of the Evaluation

Selection of the best study design in translational research is strongly influenced by the research question or purpose of the evaluation. Selection needs to be informed by previous

From clinical trials to community:
The science of translating diabetes and obesity research

research on the topic and population of interest. In many situations the goal is to select a design that will maximize generalizability and minimize bias.

Qualitative research designs, such as focus groups or structured cognitive interviews, can be particularly important sources of information if the researcher is trying to determine how best to modify an existing intervention with known effectiveness for a new setting or to enhance the cultural or demographic appropriateness of an existing intervention. Both qualitative and quantitative observational designs may be the best way to identify the most critical barriers for translating best practices into real world settings and therefore may play a critical role in intervention development.

Importance of Building on a Theoretical Framework of Behavioral Change That Is Supported by Rigorous Observational Research

The barriers to translation are multi-dimensional and complex. Therefore, interventional research designed to enhance the delivery of the highest quality of care needs to be multi-disciplinary, and because the core of the effort to improve practice is strongly linked to the behaviors of providers and patients, it should be supported by established theories of behavior change such as Social Cognitive Theory. Once a theoretical framework or conceptual model is selected, modification of the model informed by the study question and what is known from the literature become the most critical next steps. The conceptual model and the portion(s)

of the model that will be evaluated by the specific study often drive final selection of the specific design.

Nonrandomized Study Designs Are Frequently Most Appropriate for Translational Research

Although the randomized controlled trial is the strongest design to establish a causal relationship, its use in translational research is often limited by the artificial nature of the logistical constraints needed to identify and recruit participants and to conduct the trial. In translational research, there can be political, practical and ethical barriers to randomized designs. Also, because of the many multi-faceted and multi-level barriers to the delivery of health care, some of the most important questions on the translational research agenda cannot be addressed with participant-level randomized controlled trials. RCTs at the individual patient level are often not appropriate for health plan or other system level interventions. For these reasons it is critical that the translation researcher be well-versed in alternative rigorous study designs. These designs include, but are not limited to, clustered randomized trials, quasi-randomized trials with variable levels of masking, interrupted time series, observational studies with controls at a second site, and uncontrolled before and after studies. A synopsis of each of these alternate designs follows.

1. General Comment – With qualitative nonrandomized designs, the researcher may have little control over the implementation of the intervention. The strengths of nonrandomized

designs are that they are very "real world," but weaknesses include difficulty knowing what really happened and which "outcomes" are likely to have changed.

A lack of randomized control is always a threat to internal validity, but this trade-off must be placed in the context of the research question and the goals of the study.

2. Clustered Randomized Trials – Many quality improvement (QI) interventions are aimed at the provider or system level, and if you randomized at the individual patient level it is likely that there will be contamination. Randomization at higher levels will reduce this contamination but limit the power in the analyses and decrease the likelihood of detecting clinically meaningful differences in outcomes. Additionally, the risk for bias is much higher. Therefore, the overall approach should be to randomize at a higher level with as many units of randomization as the study can afford, but collect data at the patient level.

With regards to level of randomization, the lowest is the individual patient. Successively higher levels of randomization include: health care professionals; practice/hospital; provider group; health plans; and community. Lower levels of randomization increase the potential for contamination; higher levels of randomization reduce the power analysis and complicate the logistics of the implementation of the intervention(s) because potentially you may need to recruit multiple organizations to be randomized.

At higher levels of randomization, measurement of pre-intervention characteristics is important. Using these pre-intervention measurements, the researcher should consider stratification on baseline characteristics that are likely to influence the effectiveness of the intervention.

Analysis of cluster randomization should bear in mind that such randomization may violate the assumption of independence of observations within a cluster. For instance, two patients in the same practice are likely to be more similar than three from different practices. Accordingly, the researcher must estimate the intracluster correlation coefficient (ICC). There are three options to consider when analyzing data from cluster randomization trials. The first is an analysis at the cluster level uses the cluster as a unit of randomization and the unit of analysis. Each cluster is treated as one data point, which is inefficient. The second is a patient level analysis that is adjusted for variance attributable to the cluster, and the third option is a patient level analysis that allows for the correlation between clusters to be explicitly modeled. The hierarchical nature of the data is accounted for in these last two approaches.

3. Time Series Designs – Time series designs attempt to answer the question whether the intervention improves care more than the observed secular trend. They require data collection multiple times both before and after the intervention of interest so that the investigator may understand the magnitude of the secular trend. Analyses of these data must account for the auto-correlation of data collected at multiple time points. The strength of this research design is the lack of need for a control group. Its weakness is that the investigator must collect data multiple times, which may be expensive and labor intensive.

4. Controlled Before and After Designs –
This design requires the identification of a
control population with similar baseline characteristics to the intervention population. Baseline
and post-intervention data are collected on
both the control and the intervention populations, comparison of which permits identification of changes in outcomes attributable to
secular trends.

Analysis of data obtained using controlled
before and after designs is influenced by differences in baseline characteristics of the two
populations, differences can occur even in
well matched groups. Analysis of these data
should not look for significance of within group
change, as these are not appropriate and analyses must account for clustering effect by site.

5. Uncontrolled Before and After Designs –
Measurements of population characteristics
before and after a quality improvement intervention are relatively easy to collect. However,
the effect of secular trends is difficult to tease
out from changes attributable to the intervention. Accordingly, uncontrolled before and
after designs probably overestimate the benefit
derived from quality improvement interventions.

**The Need for Multi-level, Multi-factorial
Interventions To Improve Quality of Care**

It has long been recognized that the barriers
to translating high quality diabetes care to
practice settings are multi-factorial and multi-
level. Some of the most promising interventions
at the health care system and/or community-
level, such as the Chronic Care Model,
specifically address this complexity by orches-
trating change at many levels (patient, provider,
system, and community) simultaneously.
The value of this approach is that substantive
improvements in care have been documented.
But, because many organizations or communities may not have the resources to make a
variety of changes simultaneously it is critical
that collaborative research begins to identify
the relative benefits of various components
of multi-level, multi-factorial interventions.

References

Eccles M, Grimshaw J, Campbell M, Ramsay
C. Research designs for studies evaluating the
effectiveness of change and improvement strategies. *Qual Saf Health Care* 2003;12;47-52.

Garfield SA, Malozowski S, Chin MH,
Narayan KMV, Glasgow RE, Green LW,
Hiss RG, Krumholz HM, the Diabetes
Mellitus Interagency Coordinating Committee
Translation Conference Working Group.
Considerations for diabetes translational
research in real-world settings. *Diabetes
Care*, 2003; 26:2670-2674.

Hill-Briggs F. Problem solving in diabetes
self-management: a model of chronic illness
self-management behavior. *Ann Behav Med*,
2003 Summer;25(3):182-93. Review.

Wagner EH, Austin BT, Von Korff M.
Organizing care for patients with chronic illness.
Milbank Q 1996;74:511-544.

Community-Based Participatory Research for Diabetes Translation and Multi-level, Multi-factorial Interventions

Marshall H. Chin, MD, MPH

Associate Professor of Medicine; Director,
Prevention and Control Core of the
Diabetes Research and Training Center
University of Chicago

Key Points

1. We live in contexts – patients, families, providers, clinics, health systems and societies – all intertwined, all concurrent with one another. Accordingly, single focused interventions aimed at solitary targets to bring about behavior change and quality improvements will frequently have limited effects; multi-level, multi-factorial interventions are better suited to deal with complex community settings.

2. Community-based participatory research (CBPR) brings together communities, researchers and agencies collaboratively to improve health in the community. The community, researchers and agencies are equal partners, each bringing different strengths to the table.

3. Since translating and sustaining efficacious diabetes care into real-world settings requires community buy-in and individualization of interventions, CBPR efforts have significant promise.

4. CBPR may be especially useful for improving diabetes care in vulnerable, hard-to-reach populations.

Multi-level, Multi-factorial Interventions

Rationale

We live in contexts – patients, families, providers, clinics, health systems and societies – all intertwined, all concurrent with one another. Because behavior change and quality improvement activities are embedded within these several contexts, they are difficult to achieve using traditional focused interventions aimed at a solitary target. Multi-level, multi-factorial interventions are required to effect change given the complexities of relationships and contexts in real-world settings. Further, such approaches are more acceptable in these real-world settings.

Implementing a Multi-level, Multi-factorial Approach

Multi-level, multi-factorial approaches to behavior change and quality improvement activities in real-world settings requires employment of interdisciplinary and integrative teams that are respectful of one another and of the population they serve. They should define desired outcomes for each level of the complex real-world setting they are addressing and for each identifiable factor within each level.

Multi-level, multi-factorial interventions developed to achieve these outcomes should keep track of what interventions were actually done and record intermediary (successive) process variables accomplished. Studies of this type will frequently be both difficult and expensive and must bring together a variety of existing agencies and stakeholders to pool resources, commitment and energies. In contrast, a top-down approach initiated by a well-intentioned researcher will have a hard time succeeding.

Significant challenges to implementing multi-level, multi-factorial interventions exist. These include, but are not limited to: (1) determining feasibility first before full scale implementation; (2) distinguishing relative impact of each component of each intervention; (3) determining dose-response relationships; (4) needing to individualize interventions rather than employing traditional "cookie-cutter" techniques (standard product versus standard process interventions); (5) selecting appropriate statistical analytic methods, such as sample size determination and clustering effects.

Examples of Multi-level,
Multi-factorial Interventions

1. A practical model for preventing type 2 diabetes in minority youth (Burnet et al, *Diabetes Educator*, 2002) describes the relatedness of attitudinal, personal, community and environmental factors affecting behavior change in a target population.

2. A multi-level approach to diabetes in East Harlem, New York (Horowitz et al, *JGIM*, 2003) included formation of a coalition (community, providers, academics, and policy-makers), development of consensus goals of the coalition, survey of Harlem residents and creation of an infrastructure for improving diabetes care in Harlem.

Community-Based Participatory Research

Community-based participatory research (CBPR) has received increasing attention in recent years as a potential tool for translating research into practice. Nationally, much diabetes care is suboptimal and diabetes causes tremendous morbidity, some of which is preventable. Attempts to translate efficacious diabetes care into actual practice have frequently been stymied by a variety of obstacles. Some of the challenges include the need to individualize interventions to specific populations and settings, the need for community buy-in, and the difficulty of sustaining gains over time.

The crux of CBPR is a collaborative partnership among members of the community, researchers and sometimes governmental or private agencies through all phases of the research (Israel et al, *Ann. Rev. Public Health*, 1998). Community members frequently have great insight into barriers to successful diabetes care in their settings, what types of solutions might be most fruitful and how to implement and sustain an effort. CBPR may be especially promising in improving care for vulnerable and hard-to-reach populations. Researchers bring strengths in study design, data analysis, and innovative models and ideas. Agencies can help provide infrastructure and support and can facilitate dissemination and spread of successful models of care.

Challenges of CBPR

Critical challenges to performing CBPR include establishing trust among parties, defining and establishing rules of an equal partnership, sharing money and resources, and understanding each party's needs and requirements in order to create a win-win situation for all (O'Toole et al, *JGIM*, 2003). The process can be slow and trade-offs sometimes exist between an idealized, tightly controlled research environment and the practical demands of real-world people, communities and practice settings.

CBPR and Diabetes

CBPR has many potential applications for improving diabetes care and diabetes prevention. The principles of CBPR are sensible for virtually any study population and setting, but have particular relevance for diabetes. For example, the prevalence and morbidity of diabetes are especially high in minority and socioeconomically disadvantaged groups. Cultural issues are important to understand and address in providing diabetes care. In addition, diabetes prevention and treatment require community-wide efforts to prevent obesity and improve diet and exercise. If such efforts are

to be successful and sustainable, CBPR techniques and principles need to be applied.

The evaluation of diabetes care in 19 midwest community health centers (Chin et al, *Diabetes Care*, 2004) provides a demonstration of the CBPR approach to diabetes translation. The Bureau of Primary Health Care, the part of the Health Resources and Services Administration that oversees all federally funded health centers, had initiated the Health Disparities Collaborative to reduce health disparities and improve the quality of care in health centers. This initiative utilizes the Associates in Process Improvement's Model for Improvement (Langley G, et al. *The Improvement Guide: A Practical Approach to Enhancing Organizational Performance*, 1996.) and the MacColl Institute for Healthcare Innovation's Chronic Care Model (Wagner et al, *The Milbank Quarterly*, 1996). Several partners have participated in the initiative, including community health centers, the Bureau of Primary Health Care, the Agency for Healthcare Research and Quality, and the University of Chicago.

In summary, the factors impacting diabetes translational efforts in real-world settings are complex but frequently suited to CBPR principles and techniques. Successful CBPR requires expertise in the traditional methods of health services, behavioral and outcomes research in addition to skills in organizing and facilitating cross-cutting partnerships among communities, researchers, and agencies. While challenging, well-done CBPR has great promise for creating improvements in diabetes care and health that are sustainable over time.

References

Burnet D, Plaut A, Courtney R, Chin MH.
Preventing type 2 diabetes in minority youth:
A practical model and empirical evidence.
Diabetes Educator, 2002; 28:779-795.

Chin MH, Cook S, Drum ML, Jin L, Guillen M,
Humikowski CA, Koppert J, Harrison JF, Lippold
S, Schaefer CT. Improving diabetes care in
midwest community health centers with the
health disparities collaborative. *Diabetes Care*,
2004; 27 (1): 2-8.

Garfield SA, Malozowski S, Chin MH,
Narayan KMV, Glasgow RE, Green LW,
Hiss RG, Krumholz HM, the Diabetes
Mellitus Interagency Coordinating Committee
Translation Conference Working Group.
Considerations for diabetes translational
research in real-world setting. *Diabetes Care*,
2003; 26:2670-2674.

Horowitz CR, Williams L, Bickell NA.
A community-centered approach to diabetes
in East Harlem. *Journal of General Internal
Medicine*, 2003; 18:542-548.

Israel BA, Schultz AJ, Parker EA, Becker AB.
Review of community-based research:
Assessing partnership approaches to improve
public health. *Ann Rev Public Health*, 1998;
19:173-202.

Langley G, Nolan KM, Nolan TW, Norman CL,
Provost LP. The improvement guide: A practical
approach to enhancing organizational performance. *San Francisco: Jossey-Bass*, 1996.

O'Toole TP, Felix-Aaron K, Chin MH, Horowitz
CR, Tyson F. Community-based participatory
research: opportunities, challenges and
the need for a common language. *Journal of
General Internal Medicine*, 2003; 18:592-594.

Wagner EH, Austin BT, Von Korff M.
Organizing care for patients with chronic illness.
The Milbank Quarterly 1996; 74: 511-544.

Section IV

Review and Critique of Translational Research Studies

Moving Translational Research Forward: Do We Need a GPS?

Barbara K. Rimer, DrPH

Alumni Distinguished Professor of Health Behavior and Health Education
The University of North Carolina at Chapel Hill

Key Points

1. Unless there is an explicit, formal model of how dissemination fits into the scientific process, it becomes a land to which no one travels. The highest levels of the organization must recognize and reinforce the importance of dissemination or translation.

2. If we want to optimize the likelihood of dissemination or translation, we should design for it. Usually, dissemination is an afterthought.

3. *We also should create demand for dissemination.*

4. In addition, and this may be the most challenging task, we must change the culture to make dissemination research a valued area of study and attention to dissemination an expected part of the research process. The corollary of this is that there must be support for dissemination research and dissemination.

If history has taught us one thing, it is that generally health care innovations do not rapidly diffuse without special efforts. There are exceptions, but they are not the rule. And if that is true in medicine for clinical innovations, it is even truer for public health innovations. Yet, our system relies overwhelmingly on passive methods of diffusion that are ineffective.[1]

There is no bridge between discoveries and their application or even between discoveries and dissemination research.[2,3] Thus, while the U.S. has one of the best discovery engines in the world, we often fail in moving discoveries from research to practice, as several systematic reviews have shown.

It is not so much a question of us being lost as of not having a compass or global positioning system (GPS) to guide one towards the future. What do we need to find our way from discovery to delivery and from efficacy studies to effectiveness and dissemination research? We need a shared means of tracking change when we are studying it, and we need a shared means of navigating when we are driving change. The GPS system is built around a shared map and common metrics; our system should be too. My goal is to provide some rather rudimentary maps. Several coordinates are needed and we also need an overall map.

Using the diagrammed model as framework, the following sequential steps may make translation and dissemination a reality:

- Create an infrastructure for dissemination of new discoveries.
- Identify the potential universe of innovations pertinent to the discovery.
- Apply algorithms for decision-making regarding dissemination research/translation and dissemination.
- Conduct dissemination/translational research to determine best strategies for dissemination. This research should: 1) aim at understanding, influencing and/or evaluating the process of dissemination; and 2) determine what are peoples' real barriers as opposed to what they say, what really motivates them

and what will it take to overcome barriers.
- Use best strategies to disseminate selected innovations.
- Identify potential diffusion and dissemination (D&D) partners, i.e. area health education centers, schools of public health and communication, business and medical schools, health organizations, private sectors, etc.
- Disseminate the innovation/discovery using an active process through which target groups are made aware of, receive, accept and use information and other interventions. Disseminate evidence in clear actionable text to practitioners and provide economic analysis to aid program leaders in decision making.
- Evaluate efforts and provide feedback to the dissemination infrastructure where the sequence began.

A GPS for Dissemination Research (A Suggested Map)

Research funding agencies should have explicit models that include translation/dissemination as territories to be expanded. At the National Cancer Institute (*http://dccps.nci.nih.gov*), we adapted a model from the National Cancer Institute of Canada (see diagram below) to recognize explicitly and to demonstrate in resource allocation the important role of dissemination in moving discoveries from discovery to delivery. *Unless there is an explicit, formal model of how dissemination fits into the scientific process, it becomes a land to which no one travels. The highest levels of the organization must recognize and reinforce the importance of dissemination or translation.*

ROLE OF DISSEMINATION CORE IN RESEARCH LIFECYCLE

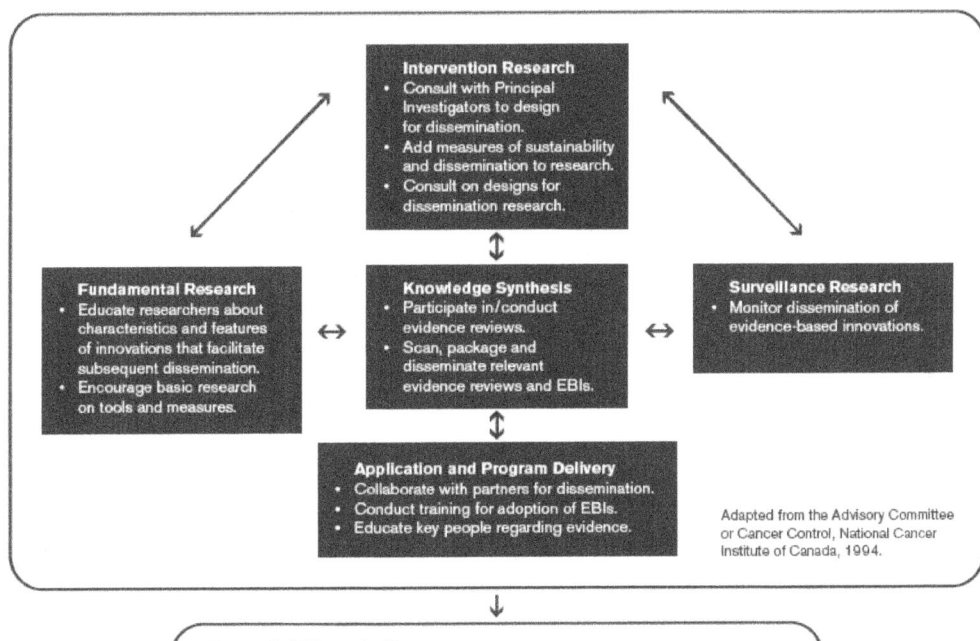

Intervention Research
- Consult with Principal Investigators to design for dissemination.
- Add measures of sustainability and dissemination to research.
- Consult on designs for dissemination research.

Fundamental Research
- Educate researchers about characteristics and features of innovations that facilitate subsequent dissemination.
- Encourage basic research on tools and measures.

Knowledge Synthesis
- Participate in/conduct evidence reviews.
- Scan, package and disseminate relevant evidence reviews and EBIs.

Surveillance Research
- Monitor dissemination of evidence-based innovations.

Application and Program Delivery
- Collaborate with partners for dissemination.
- Conduct training for adoption of EBIs.
- Educate key people regarding evidence.

Adapted from the Advisory Committee or Cancer Control, National Cancer Institute of Canada, 1994.

Research & Dissemination
- Consult with researchers regarding designs and measures for dissemination research.
- Provide support for pilot dissemination research.
- Package interventions for dissemination research and dissemination.

Why Does Dissemination Not Occur Routinely?

The literature shows that there are many reasons for the failure of dissemination.[1,4] Some of the earlier speakers addressed barriers, such as lack of time, failure of the intended users to perceive the "innovation" as truly useful, and many other reasons. My 20+ years as a researcher convince me that a large part of the reason is that we do not *design* for dissemination. Thus, the probability of successful dissemination is very low from the outset of discovery. The rewards for researchers, the grants process, the selection process for who becomes a successful researcher militate against interventions that are designed for sustainability. *If we want to optimize the likelihood of dissemination or translation, we should design for it.*

Creating New Interventions – The Art and Science of Dissemination (Translational) Research

There are some effective interventions (e.g., reminders and brief counseling); some regimens for weight loss (e.g., Diabetes Prevention Program protocol); and combinations of cognitive behavioral therapy (CBT) and education. However, they are underused in practice, and

From clinical trials to community:
The science of translating diabetes and obesity research

there are not enough of them. As a general rule, we should design the simplest effective intervention, not the most complex. To do this, use an adaptive step design to identify the minimum intervention needed for change (MINC).

Effective interventions communicate to practitioners what are core immutable aspects of interventions and what elements can be adapted locally. Interventions should encourage partnerships between researchers, practitioners and people with skills in dissemination. These partnerships are developed through interpersonal links, as Huberman[5] pointed out, spread through the life of a given study. Such links allow nonresearchers to find their niche and their voice while a study is still young and promote a conversation among professionals, each bringing different expertise to bear on the same topic. Authors should report sufficient detail about their interventions to enable readers to understand what was actually done. In this way, a positive interventional experience can be reproduced with other populations at other sites.

How Can We Change the Pace of Dissemination?

We should take more of an engineering approach to the problem, designing for dissemination from the discovery phase, working at the outset in partnership with potential adopters for reality testing, and creating agency models that facilitate and reward dissemination in explicit ways. In addition, and this may be the most challenging task, we must change the culture to make dissemination research a valued area of study and attention to dissemination an expected part of the research process. This might include creating knowledge teams within agencies that conduct knowledge syntheses and identify interventions/innovations that are ready for dissemination as well as areas that need further research. It also should include grant support for dissemination research and production support for turning discoveries into products and practices. Both scientists and government often stop once the discovery has been made and shown to be effective. That is no longer adequate.

We Should Create Demand for Dissemination

Traditionally, there has not been a constituency for many innovations, especially those in the behavioral and social sciences. The synergistic model developed by the RWJF and the NIH's Office of Behavioral and Social Sciences Research (see diagram on next page) highlights the importance of creating the demand side of the picture.

Some Areas Are New Lands and Need Special Assistance To Develop

This seems especially true for innovations in the behavioral and social sciences. Because most of these innovations won't hold great promise for generating profits, they are likely to be underdeveloped lands. Thus, it behooves us to develop the infrastructure to facilitate dissemination research and dissemination. Failure to do this will result in continued diminution of our capacity to improve the population's health.

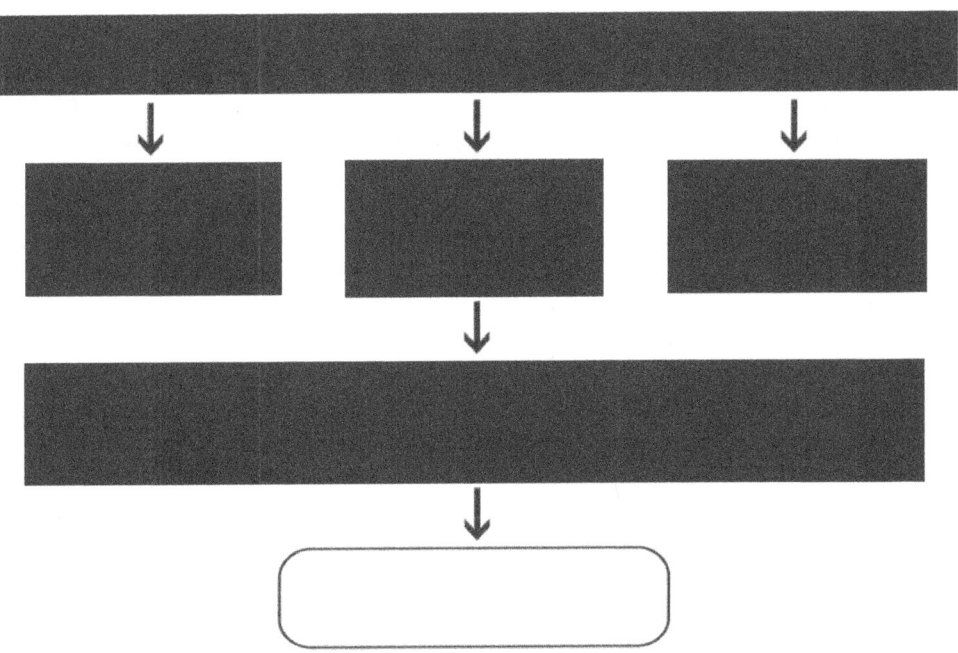

References

1. Bero LA, Grilli R, Grimshaw JM, Harvey E, Oxman AD, Thomson MA. Closing the gap between research and practice: An overview of systematic reviews of interventions to promote the implementation of research findings. The Cochrane Effective Practice and Organization of Care Review Group. *BMJ*, 1998;317(7156):465-468.

2. Hiatt RA, Rimer BK. A new strategy for cancer control research. *Cancer Epidemiol Biomarkers Prev*, 1999;8(11):957-964.

3. Ellis P, Robinson P, Ciliska D, Armour T, Raina P, Brouwers M et al. *Diffusion and Dissemination of Evidence-based Cancer Control Interventions. Evidence Report/ Technology Assessment Number 79.* Rockville, MD: Agency for Healthcare Research and Quality, 2003.

4. Glasgow RE, Lichtenstein E, Marcus AC. Why don't we see more translation of health promotion research to practice? Rethinking the efficacy-to-effectiveness transition. *Am J Public Health*, 2003;93(8):1261-1267.

5. Huberman M. Research utilization: The state of the art. Knowledge and policy. *The International Journal of Knowledge Transfer and Utilization*, 1994; 7:13-33.

Perspective of NIH Review Committees

Alan M. Delamater, PhD

Professor of Pediatrics and Psychology
University of Miami School of Medicine

Key Points

1. The proposed intervention must address a significant public health issue and have a solid empirical basis in efficacy studies.

2. The study approach should be directed to diverse populations; conducted in real-world settings; have an appropriate control group; use an intent-to-treat design; provide measures of implementation, including process measures such as treatment fidelity, staffing time and costs, and consumer and staff satisfaction; and include reliable, valid and clinically practical measures of both short and long-term outcomes, including health behaviors, health outcomes and quality of life. The intervention approach should be well described, innovative, and have a theoretical basis, and the study design should include measurement of hypothesized mediators of treatment response.

3. The investigators must have established a collaboration with the community-based organization, have expertise with the proposed intervention, and have demonstrated that the approach is feasible in the proposed setting.

4. The intervention approach must have a high degree of external validity, with high potential of being translated into other settings.

Importance of the Issue and Efficacy of the Intervention Approach

The first concern of the reviewer is that the investigators have proposed a study of high public health significance, one that is likely to advance the state of scientific knowledge and have an influence on clinical practice. Assuming this is the case, it is essential that the intervention approach proposed be one that already has been shown to be efficacious. In the cycle of clinical research, interventions must be shown to have efficacy under controlled conditions. That is, under ideal conditions, the intervention has a significant positive health impact. When this has been demonstrated, the next phase of research is to test the effectiveness of the intervention in real-world settings with diverse patient populations.

Key Elements of the Study Approach

In order for an intervention to be translatable, it must be demonstrated to be effective in real-world clinical settings in the community. Therefore, a key element of the study approach is that it is targeted to a patient population that is commonly seen in such settings. The patient population is likely to have one or more comorbidities; thus, the inclusion and exclusion criteria may be less stringent than in efficacy studies. The sampling and randomization plans

From clinical trials to community:
The science of translating diabetes and obesity research

should be clearly described. Among the important design issues to consider are the nature of the control group and the statistical analyses to be employed. In efficacy research, where internal validity is very important, there is typically more experimental control. For example, a control group often is equated to the experimental group in terms of contact with the health care team. In effectiveness and translational research, the control group should be one with ecological validity – e.g., usual or enhanced clinical care – even though strict control for attention and contact may not be achieved. The statistical design should include an intent-to-treat analysis, with careful documentation of the number and percentage of patients who did not complete the proposed treatment, the reasons for not completing, as well as methods for handling missing data in the data analysis.

Process measures of the intervention are essential, including measurement of treatment implementation (i.e., fidelity), the costs of providing the treatment, and satisfaction of patients receiving the intervention as well as staff who provide it. The intervention itself should be clearly specified, innovative, and described in a way that it could be replicable. Another important consideration is who will provide the intervention, whether they will be research staff or existing staff of the agency who have been trained by the research staff. In efficacy studies, research staff may be essential to provide the intervention while in translational studies existing agency staff should be trained to provide the intervention.

The proposed plan for outcomes assessment should include a variety of reliable and valid measures that have clinical utility. If such measures are not practical and cannot be routinely employed in community settings, they likely would create too great a burden for patients, leading to attrition. Besides measurement of relevant health behaviors and health outcomes, quality of life should also be included as a key patient outcome. The proposed intervention approach should have a well-specified theoretical basis, and hypothesized mediators of treatment should be included in the assessment and data analysis plan.

Collaboration, Expertise, and Feasibility

The investigators must have clearly established collaborative relationships with the participating community-based clinics or agencies. Letters of agreement from community leaders to the principal investigator are essential to document that collaborative arrangements have been achieved. The investigative team should be interdisciplinary, have a track record of publications and grants relevant to the proposed study aims and procedures, and be in an institutional environment likely to facilitate achievement of the study aims. The investigators should have conducted pilot tests in the community settings with the proposed study population in order to demonstrate that the study approach is feasible.

External Validity and Translation

Potential for translation is a very significant concern for the reviewer. To what patient populations and settings are the study findings expected to generalize to? External validity is key to translation; the proposed study should be designed with this factor in mind. Transferability (i.e., application to diverse settings) depends upon well-specified description of the intervention approach (including treatment manuals and staff training), and evidence that the intervention leads to maintenance of change over a reasonably long period of follow-up – not only for patients, but also for the setting in terms of its system of health care delivery. Barriers to successful implementation should be documented in both the short and long-term. Translation is likely after successful demonstration of long-term effectiveness with a diverse patient population in a real-world clinical setting.

Summary of Reviewers Concerns

- Importance of the issue.
- Soundness of the approach – recruitment and retention of diverse study sample; type, delivery and translatability of proposed intervention; measurement of process, outcome, and mediator variables; use of theory; appropriate design; convincing power analysis and statistical plan.
- Pilot studies to demonstrate feasibility.
- Collaborative arrangements with community-based clinics.
- Experience of the team.

References

Garfield SA et al. Considerations for diabetes translational research in real-world settings. *Diabetes Care*, 2003; 26: 2670-2674.

Glasgow RE. Translating research to practice: Lessons learned, areas for improvement, and future directions. *Diabetes Care*, 2003; 26: 2451-2456.

Moher D et al. The CONSORT Statement: Revised recommendations for improving the quality of reports of parallel-group randomized trials. *JAMA*, 2001; 285: 1987-1991.

Venkat Narayan KM et al. Translation research for chronic disease: The case for diabetes. *Diabetes Care*, 2000; 23: 1794-1798.

Translational Research: The Medical Editor's View

Harold C. Sox, MD, MACP

Editor
Annals of Internal Medicine

Key Points

1. Medical journals play an essential role in the evaluation and dissemination of clinical research.

2. The process of scientific review and editing is costly.

3. The open access model of medical journalism provides free access to content and passes the cost of review from the subscriber to the author. This model is unproven but currently under test.

4. Publishing unbiased information about the effectiveness of new technology serves the interests of the public but is difficult to achieve.

The Role of Journals in the Advance of Medical Science

Medical journals play two indispensable roles in the advance of medical science. The first is peer review, whereby an author's scientific peers evaluate the research. For research submitted to clinical journals, their criteria center on judgments about its internal and external validity, its novelty, and its potential impact on patient care. If an article is accepted for publication, the author and the journal enter into a partnership that is both antagonistic and cooperative. It is antagonistic because the journal almost always wants the author to do more to buttress the internal validity of the research. It is cooperative because both parties want the same thing: a transparent account of the methods and the findings and a balanced discussion of the significance of the research and its strengths and weaknesses.

The second role is dissemination of the research findings to the research community, the clinical community, and the public at large. The process of dissemination also elevates the status of the research. A finding that has "passed peer review" occupies a state that is much closer to "the truth" than a finding that has not. Members of the public assume that published research is the truth, and it's likely that many physicians, too busy keeping up with clinical duties to read research articles critically, rely on journals to tell them the truth.

Peer Review: Imperfect but Indispensable and Costly

Peer review maximizes the probability that an article tells the unbiased truth, but it is not perfect, as research has shown. Still, it is the best way we have to protect the public interest. The peer review process is partly external. The journal sends the article to experts in the topic, and they comment on validity, novelty, and potential impact, and they suggest ways to improve the report. Most reviewers spend three hours or more on a review, and a three page review is common. The reviews influence the decision to publish an article, but they are advisory to the editors. The decision to publish is just the beginning of peer review, since the editors are typically very experienced at evaluating manuscripts and ask the authors to make many substantial changes beyond those suggested in the reviewers' comments. In addition, most major journals include statisticians among their editorial team. Statistical review may reveal fatal flaws in an article and typically asks for refinements in the statistical analysis. All these people cost money, and a major clinical journal may have an editorial budget of $15,000 to $20,000 per original research article published. Subscription fees, advertising income, sales of reprints, and membership dues (if a professional organization sponsors the journal) are the major sources of income to offset these expenses.

Manuscript Review Issues

Editorial Decision Criteria

Editors of general medical journals (such as the Annals of Internal Medicine) base their decision to publish a manuscript on three criteria: 1) Does the evidence support the conclusions? ("is it true?"); 2) How does it advance the field? ("is it new?"); 3) How will it affect patient care?

Is It True?

External validity: to whom and to what do the conclusions apply? Describe how the study cohort was formed – population to be studied, recruiting, inclusion and exclusion criteria. A figure to describe cohort formation is often useful. Describe the intervention carefully. Be clear on what the study is to prove. For an efficacy study, does the intervention work? For an effectiveness study, does it work in the real world?

Internal validity: do the data support the conclusions? State clearly the primary hypothesis and outcome measures and distinguish these from

secondary hypothesis and exploratory analysis. Account for loss of patients. Adjust for known confounders and test the effects of potential unmeasured confounding (sensitivity analysis).

"Negative" versus "inconclusive" studies: the point estimate of the outcome in a negative study has no important effect and the 95% confidence interval for effect size does not include a clinically important effect. An "inconclusive" study has no important effect, but the 95% confidence interval for effect size does include a clinically important effect.

Avoid a biased presentation or interpretation: give a balanced account of the findings and their implications; employ a cautious tone; let the findings speak for themselves and don't exaggerate claims of clinical effect or publication priority.

Address the possibility of bias in the presentation or interpretation: for sponsored research, state clearly who is responsible for the design and conduct of the study, the manuscript, and the decision to publish; declare conflicts of interest.

Is It New?

In the introduction section of the manuscript, establish the context of the study being reported and show clearly the gap that the research will fill.

In the discussion section of the manuscript, state early and clearly how the principal finding advances the field. Cite the findings of previous work and consider using an evidence table to summarize previous work and yours. Be sure to discuss the limitations of the study.

Common Shortcomings

- Inadequate description of cohort assembly.
- Failure to involve a statistician from the very beginning.
- Underpowered.
- Single site.
- Inattention to costs of intervention.

Common Statistical Errors

- Calling an inconclusive study "negative."
- Unstable predictive models: too many predictive variables for the number of outcome events.
- Combining heterogeneous studies in a meta-analysis.
- Step-wise addition of variables to regression model.
- Biased methods for dealing with missing values.
- Not adjusting for clustering by physician or clinic.
- Not taking into account measurement error.
- Adjusting only for baseline values of covariates that change over time.

Summary of Factors That Lead to Acceptance

- Hot topic.
- High impact disease.
- Unexpected but believable findings.
- First report.
- Large effect size, narrow confidence interval.
- Complements recently accepted article.
- A good vehicle for an editorial on an important subject.
- High level of public interest in topic.

Summary of Factors That Lead to Rejection

- Fatal flaw.
- Many nonfatal problems with study design and execution.

- Secondary report of major study that adds little new information.
- Nothing to distinguish it from previous work on the topic.
- Small effect size, wide confidence interval.
- Hot issue but recently resolved.
- The journal has already published a lot on this topic recently.

What Else do Editors Like To See?

- A diverse study population that represents the world of clinical practice; multi-center studies (after adjusting for center effect) are stronger than single center studies.
- A large study population; which narrows confidence intervals, reduces the risk of false-negative or false-positive conclusions, and permits powerful sub-group analyses.

Additional Editorial Suggestions

- Consider how the study might influence health policy.
- Do cost-effectiveness analysis.
- Use decision analysis to set target enrollment and choose the key questions to study.
- Consider alternatives to randomized controlled trials.
- Do studies of chronic disease.
- Characterize patient preferences for the outcomes that they might experience.

Writing Style Suggestions

- Use short declarative sentences and the active voice.
- Paragraph structure: The topic sentence should state briefly what the paragraph is about. The final sentence should provide a transition to the next paragraph.

- Be concise.
- Avoid inflaming reviewers and editors.
- In the discussion section, discuss how your paper adds to prior work and the limitations of the research.

The Open Access Model of Medical Journalism

The first experiment in open access medical journalism began when the British Medical Journal made all of its material available on-line at no cost to anyone. The BMJ announced this year that they would end the experiment after ten years because of falling institutional subscription rates. The most interesting new development in medical journalism is the publishing model adopted by the Public Library of Science. This journal, which currently competes with journals like Science, Nature, and Cell for manuscripts, provides free access to its article from the day of publication. It reduces expenses by publishing only electronically, and in lieu of subscription fees, it charges the authors a publication fee, which currently is $1500 per article published.

Publishing Unbiased Information About the Effectiveness of New Technology Serves the Interests of the Public but Is Difficult To Achieve

Commercial companies often do clinical trials that compare a new product to the current standard of care or a placebo intervention. These trials typically involve many sites of care. The authors are usually well-known leaders in the topic area, usually writing on behalf of a larger group of participating physicians. These individuals enter into a contract with the com-mercial company, often a pharmaceutical manu-facturer. The contract specifies the conditions of the trial and the roles and rights of the authors and other participating physicians.

Too often, the participating physicians have had limited roles in designing the study and analyz-ing the results. Too often, they have not had the right to see all of the data. Too often, the deci-sion to publish has rested, by contract, with the sponsor. Too often, the company has drafted the article. Too often, the authors did not enjoy the independence that the public attributes to a scientist. To address this subject, each of a group of large, general medical journals pub-lished a jointly written editorial in September 2001. The message was simple. These journals would require the corresponding author of an article to attest that he or she (speaking on behalf of the participating scientists) had an important role in study design, had access to the data, had an important role in the analysis of the study data, and a controlling interest in the content of the article and the decision to publish it. The effects of this joint action are known only anecdotally, and control of the data remains an important unresolved question.

Reference

Davidoff F, DeAngelis CD, Drazen JM, Hoey J, Hojgaard L, Horton R, Kotzin S,Nicholls MG, Nylenna M, Overbeke AJ, Sox HC, Van der Weyden MB, Wilkes MS. Sponsorship, author-ship, and accountability. *Ann Intern Med*. 2001 Sep 18;135(6):463-6. (This editorial appeared in all of the journals represented by the authors of the editorial).

The Outlook for Translational Research

Translating the Diabetes Prevention Program

David G. Marrero, PhD

Professor of Medicine, Director,
Diabetes Prevention and Control Center
Indiana University School of Medicine

Key Points

1. The DPP demonstrated that type 2 diabetes can be delayed or possibly prevented by lifestyle modification and use of medication. The interventions, however, were not designed in a way that is directly deliverable on a public health scale.

2. Translation on a public health scale will require:

- Increased community awareness of risk factors for diabetes and strategies for reducing them;
- Defining real-world strategies to identify individuals at risk who are likely to benefit most from lifestyle modification;
- Developing intervention strategies to enhance dissemination and sustainability in nonresearch environments, particularly community venues where it can be accessed by broader segments of the population.

Delaying or Preventing Type 2 Diabetes: The Diabetes Prevention Program Experience

The Diabetes Prevention Program (DPP) demonstrated that an intensive lifestyle intervention involving weight loss and exercise and the use of select medications may delay or prevent the development of type 2 diabetes in those at high risk.[1] The lifestyle program used by the DPP was not designed, however, in a way that is directly deliverable on a public health scale. The DPP study was an efficacy trial using resource-intensive strategies to achieve intervention delivery and to maintain adherence.[1, 2] The two major goals of the lifestyle intervention were loss and maintenance of 7% of body mass and participation in at least 150 minutes per week of moderate intensity physical activities. To achieve these goals, each participant was assigned a case manager, or "lifestyle coach," who delivered the 16-session behavioral core curriculum, monitored maintenance, and provided ongoing support on a one-on-one basis. The behavioral core curriculum was offered and closely supervised in only select DPP clinical centers. Coaches were registered dieticians or had at least a Master's degree in fields of exercise physiology, behavioral psychology, or health education, and they were provided with substantial resources for incentivizing participants to maintain behavioral goals.

Creating Increased Public Awareness

If a diabetes prevention effort geared toward weight loss and physical activity is to be feasible on a public health scale, we first need to raise public awareness of risk factors for developing diabetes and potential ways to reduce risk. This will require a mixture of community-based, multimedia communications targeting persons at risk. This process has already started with the introduction of the Small Steps, Big Rewards PSA series by the National Diabetes Education Program. In addition, increased communication needs to be directed towards health care providers to make them aware of modifiable risk factors, strategies for identifying persons at increased risk, and how they may assist these individuals to initiate risk reducing behaviors. One example is the NDEP toolkit for primary care physicians.

Developing Interventions Suitable for the Public Health Sector

To translate the DPP into the public sector, it is necessary to develop strategies that can be tailored to meet the diverse needs of varied populations in a broad range of communities. In this context, we must begin to consider several issues inherent to the translation of a successful clinical program that was designed for efficacy. These issues include:

1. Defining Real-World Strategies To Identify Individuals at Risk Who are Likely to Benefit Most From Lifestyle Modification.

Identifying high-risk individuals who meet the DPP study's criterion of impaired glucose tolerance (IGT) is a complex translational issue. Several models have been proposed, however, there are unique barriers for applying each strategy in different screening environments. Healthcare settings are uniquely suited to screen for IGT in patients with a number of other risk criteria.[3] In such settings, the ultimate screening goal may involve definitive oral glucose tolerance testing to discriminate true IGT from both transient impaired fasting glucose and actual type 2 diabetes. An OGT may be costly, but could lead to considerably higher predictive value, compared to less intensive approaches. However, this approach restricts availability of risk screening only to persons with regular access to a healthcare system. In addition, screening efforts that are isolated within discreet healthcare environments may not identify and refer a large enough at-risk population to justify the up-front costs of marketing, implementing, and maintaining a lifestyle modification program in the community.

In contrast, community-based strategies for identifying individuals at high-risk for diabetes can be limited by several factors, such as lower feasibility for obtaining laboratory-based assessments or for using complex calculations that incorporate a combination of questionnaire and laboratory data.[4] These limitations can lead to considerable misclassification of disease risk, particularly in unselected community populations.[4-7] In addition, screening outside healthcare settings may be less effective because of difficulties in arranging appropriate follow-up testing or care after an "abnormal" screen.[4] However, despite these limitations, a carefully designed and selective community-based screening approach may be essential for reaching a broader segment of the at-risk population that has limited access to particular local healthcare systems with screening efforts.

2. Adapting Program Format To Enhance Dissemination and Sustainability in Nonresearch Environments.

An important translational issue is whether modifications in the DPP program format to improve the feasibility for offering community settings will alter the outcomes. Changes studied to date include: 1) shifting the core curriculum delivery format from a one-on-one to a group-based setting; 2) shortening the duration of the core curriculum period to decrease participant time burden; and 3) eliminating costly incentives used to enhance subject performance. Changes that are introduced need to be supported by research demonstrating that the success of behavioral weight loss strategies are enhanced when individuals are trained in behavioral concepts such as problem solving, social support, goal-setting, stimulus control, and self-monitoring.[8,9]

3. Exploring Program Delivery in Community Venues Where It Can Be Accessed by Broader Segments of the Population.

It is particularly essential to consider implementation models that do not restrict program access only to patients of healthcare systems, thereby discounting a greater population that is otherwise "healthy." This suggests that the success of a translation model requires involvement by a community organization that is committed to investing resources to improve community health and is experienced in implementing sustainable versions of beneficial health and wellness programs that were conceived from science. Examples of such organizations include the YMCA, the Boys and Girls Clubs of America, and Parks and Recreation Departments. Such models will need to investigate issues inherent in the community such as cost recovery, staffing, and sustainability. Overcoming these barriers will require considerable translational research, not just for the DPP but all intensive community-based diabetes programs.

References

1. Knowler WC, Barrett-Connor E, Fowler SE, et al. Reduction in the incidence of type 2 diabetes with lifestyle intervention or metformin. *N Engl J Med.* Feb 7 2002; 346(6):393-403.

2. The Diabetes Prevention Program (DPP): description of lifestyle intervention. *Diabetes Care.* Dec 2002;25(12):2165-2171.

3. Screening for type 2 diabetes. *Diabetes Care.* Jan 2003;26 Suppl 1:S21-24.

4. Engelgau MM, Narayan KM, Herman WH. Screening for type 2 diabetes. *Diabetes Care.* Oct 2000;23(10):1563-1580.

5. Sherwin RS, Anderson RM, Buse JB, et al. The prevention or delay of type 2 diabetes. *Diabetes Care.* Jan 2003;26 Suppl 1:S62-69.

6. Rolka DB, Narayan KM, Thompson TJ, et al. Performance of recommended screening tests for undiagnosed diabetes and dysglycemia. *Diabetes Care.* Nov 2001;24(11):1899-1903.

7. Engelgau MM, Narayan KM. Finding undiagnosed type 2 diabetes: Is it worth the effort? *Eff Clin Pract.* Nov-Dec 2001;4(6):281-283.

8. Jakicic JM, Clark K, Coleman E, et al. American College of Sports Medicine position stand. Appropriate intervention strategies for weight loss and prevention of weight regain for adults. *Med Sci Sports Exerc.* Dec 2001;33(12):2145-2156.

9. *Clinical guidelines on the identification, evaluation, and treatment of overweight and obesity in adults.* Bethesda, MD: National Heart, Lung, and Blood Institute; National Institutes of Health; Public Health Service; September 1998 1998. 98-4083.

Translating Obesity and Diabetes Research: Some Challenges and Recommendations

Ken Resnicow, PhD

School of Public Health
University of Michigan

Problems/Challenges

1. Disconnect between research interventions and clinical practice.

2. Formidable practitioner and system barriers to effective treatment.

Solutions/Recommendations

1. Recast obesity as a behavioral rather than medical condition: Flip the nexus of care to behavioral professionals.

2. Recast obesity as a cluster of heterogeneous conditions: Consider the OBESITIES.

Disconnect Between Research Interventions and Clinical Practice

Many of the strategies and programs recommended for the clinical management of obesity were developed and tested under efficacy conditions.[1,2] Under these circumstances, interventions are generally delivered by highly skilled practitioners, who typically receive extensive training and supervision. The extent to which research-based interventions can be replicated under real world conditions remains unclear. Moreover, whereas the primary "gatekeepers" for detection and treatment of obesity appear to be primary care physicians, many (if not most) of the successful interventions were conducted by psychologists or behavioral specialists. Physicians often lack the training, skills, and confidence required to implement the behavioral strategies required to effectively modify diet and physical activity.[3] As a result obesity remains under, if not mistreated, in clinical practice. More research is needed to develop and test interventions that a priori are designed for delivery by physicians that account for limitations of medical training, its implicit orientation, practice structure, and reimbursement guidelines.

Formidable Practitioner and System Barriers to Effective Treatment

Successful obesity treatment often requires interventions of considerable intensity, duration and frequency that is beyond that available in traditional medical practice. Additionally, medical practices (and practitioners) are often not equipped to conduct many of the recommended strategies such as family and/or group meetings, stress management, and behavioral counseling. Practice guidelines for pediatric and adult obesity management include referral to behavioral and/or dietetic counselors. Whereas such support may be available in academic medical centers, the extent to which community-based medical practices have access to these resources is unclear. Without such supportive services the impact of treatment may be considerably attenuated.

Increasingly obesity has been conceptualized as a chronic condition requiring long-term disease management similar to clinical models used to guide diabetes and hypertension care. Whereas adoption of the disease management model may be helpful as it can encourage physicians to be diligent and proactive in their monitoring and treatment of obese patients, there is also concern that this model may lead to an overemphasis on pharmacologic treatment and the medical risk factors associated with obesity and a de-emphasis on the underlying behavioral and social etiologies.

Recast Obesity as a Behavioral Rather than Medical Condition: Flip the Nexus of Care to Behavioral Professionals

"To treat malaria, go to a physician.
To prevent it, consult a mosquito controller."

Documenting the severe medical consequences of obesity is essential for motivating patients, practitioners, and policy makers to attend to the epidemic. However, despite its numerous and severe physiologic medical sequellae, the origins of obesity (and the recent increase in its prevalence) are largely social and behavioral. This raises questions about our current treatment paradigm. The medical profession has been (perhaps de facto, rather than by design) designated as the primary gatekeepers charged with stemming the epidemic. In the current model, behavioral and nutritional professions have largely been cast as second-

ary resources; as treatment adjuncts. This has considerable implications for how we conceptualize obesity and how we reimburse those who care for it. Given the behavioral origins of the condition, perhaps we should reconsider the nexus of professional responsibility. A model that casts behavioral professionals as the first line in clinical care would be more consistent with the underlying etiology. This paradigm shift however, would require dramatic alterations in how managed care reimburses behavioral counseling, including a de-emphasis on the co-morbidities of obesity and a greater focus on the underlying behavioral and psychologic causes as well as alteration for how the public perceives the role of behavioral and psychologic professions. *As part of this reconceptualization, individuals, rather than being viewed as suffering from obesity, might be seen as having a particular eating or activity problem. Obesity becomes the symptom rather than the disease.*

Creation of an obesity treatment sub-specialty within psychology and/or health education not unlike what has been done with HIV and substance use specialists, should be considered.

Recast Obesity as a Cluster of Heterogeneous Conditions: Consider the OBESITIES.

Perhaps like cancer, obesity should be considered not as one disease but a rubric of many diseases, each with a unique etiology, course, and treatment. As noted by Epstein:[4] "Treating obesity as a homogenous condition, with all participants receiving a common intervention, might contribute to the mixed treatment outcomes that are reported (page 566)". Factors operative in obesity include: age, gender, dietary patterns, physical activity, socioeconomics, psychosocial issues, metabolism, co-morbidities, familial/genetic determinants and race/ethnicity/cultural characteristics. With each of these factors having a greater or lesser influence on obesity on an individual case, classification and subclassification schemes should be developed to adequately describe the heterogeneity of the obesities.

The reasons for energy imbalance can be highly variable across individuals, and treatment programs can be better tailored to these individual differences. For example, excess caloric intake could be due to consuming high fat foods or foods high in simple carbohydrates. And for some "high-fat" food consumers, excess caloric intake could be attributed to one or two foods, while for others excess intake could be attributed to a variety of foods. In addition to focusing of specific foods, tailoring could also account for eating patterns such as consuming large serving sizes, rapid eating, eating second helpings, or eating at "all you can eat" establishments. The same applies to activity patterns. Despite the numerous potential differences in behavioral patterns, our current detection and treatment algorithms often fail to account for such micro-level individual differences. As noted above, regardless of etiology, patients are given an identical diagnosis and often identical treatment.

Individualizing treatment (and diagnosis) could also address genetic and metabolic characteristics. For example, individuals with low resting metabolism or thermogenic response to food may require unique interventions. Interventions could also be tailored according to family factors. For example, youth with two overweight parents may require different intervention than youth with two lean parents, while youth with psychologically high- functioning parents may require different treatment than those with parental psychopathology.

References

1. Barlow SE, Dietz WH. Obesity evaluation and treatment: Expert committee recommendations. *Pediatrics* 1998; 102(3):e29-.

2. Grizzard T. Undertreatment of obesity. *JAMA*. 2002;288(17):2177.

3. NIH-NHLBI and the North American Association for the study of obesity. *The practical guide: Identification, evaluation, and treatment of overweight and obesity in adults*: NIH, Pub Number 00-4084; 2000.

4. Epstein L, Myers M, Raynor H, Saelens B. Treatment of pediatric obesity. *Pediatrics* 1998;101(3):554-70.

Changing Practices/Changing Lives:
The Health Disparities Collaboratives Bringing Science to Life

David M. Stevens, MD, MA

Senior Medical Officer for Quality Improvement
Center for Quality Improvement and Patient Safety
Agency for Healthcare Research and Quality

Key Points

1. System change is necessary to translate science into clinical practice.

2. Implementing, spreading and sustaining positive system change in health centers supports the need to address leadership, to transform clinical systems through a model of care and to apply strategies for learning and improvement. This systematic approach addresses formal, informal, and technical aspects of care and organizational and personal behavior.

3. Infrastructure and partnerships at the practice, state and national level are essential to implement, support, sustain and spread positive change.

4. Although the methods of science and those of quality improvement are different, a continual dynamic interaction between them facilitates the growth of knowledge, its timely adoption and the generation of new questions to be studied. Research methods need to address complex systems and not solely rely on understanding a system by splitting it into its component pieces.

Background

As part of the DHHS strategy towards eliminating health disparities among Americans, the HRSA/Bureau of Primary Health Care is implementing a major initiative, the Health Disparities Collaboratives (HDC) in HRSA-supported, private not-for-profit health centers. Health Centers serve 10.3 million underserved and racially and ethnically diverse populations, with over 900 community controlled comprehensive primary care health center organizations throughout the nation. The Collaboratives represent a four-prong strategy that addresses senior leadership, implements a care model by utilizing improvement and learning models to change practice, supports an infrastructure to support and sustain improvement, and develops partnerships at the local and national level. The care model is a population-based care model pioneered by Edward Wagner, M.D. at the MacColl Institute for Healthcare Innovation and supported by the Robert Wood Johnson Foundation (see references 2 and 3). It consists of six basic elements: patient self-management, clinical decision support, delivery system re-design, clinical information system, organizational leadership and strong partnerships with local government and community organizations. The learning model is based on the Institute for Healthcare Improvement's "Breakthrough Series." The improvement model is a rapid approach to accelerate system change developed by Associates in Process Improvement.

Health Centers participate in yearlong intense learning and improvement activities that involve attending three learning sessions and a final congress sharing the improvement tests, changes and documented results accomplished at the health center level. This is followed by continued improvement activities, continual reporting of nationally shared measures and dissemination of the successful changes made to the delivery system. A national and regional/state infrastructure based in the Primary Care Associations supports the Health Centers quality improvement work, including the spread and sustaining of positive system changes.

Major Accomplishments

Over 500 Health Centers are participating in the Health Disparities Collaboratives generating major documented improvements in diabetes, depression, cardiovascular, cancer, and asthma care for over 160,000 patients. Depression screening is integrated into all the current chronic care collaboratives as well. A pilot to apply HDC models to prevention, including obesity, is currently underway.

There are five diabetes core measures (Table 1), and additional measures focused on preventing complications (Table 2). Table 3 summarizes core outcomes for health centers participating in the HDC for persons in health center diabetes registries in January 2001 and for persons in health center diabetes registries in October 2003.

Table 1. Diabetes Core Measures 2003-2004

- Average HbA1c.
- Two HbA1cs, at least 3 months apart, in last year.
- Documentation of self-management goal setting.
- Cardiac risk reduction: ACE/ARB and statins.
- Dental exam if health center has a dental practice.

Table 2. Diabetes Additional Measures 2003-2004

- Depression screening in past 12 months.
- Patients with LDL <100.
- ASA or other antithrombotic agent.
- Current smokers.
- Dilated eye exam.
- Foot exam.
- Microalbuminuria screening in past year.
- Vaccination: influenza, pneumococcal.
- Dental exam in last year.

Table 3. Core Outcomes for Health Centers

Measure	January 2001	October 2003
Number of Health Centers	88	300
1. Number of persons with DM in registries	13,387	88,854
2. Two HbA1cs per year, at least 3 months apart	55.8% (7,470 Patients)	36% (31,987 Patients)
3. Documented Patient Self-Management Goal	39% (5,221 Patients)	40% (35,542 Patients)
4. Average HbA1c	8.46%	8.00%

Partnerships formed at the national, state and community levels have resulted in increased access to expertise and resources. Through the partnership with CDC, there are 39 CDC-sponsored state health department diabetes programs trained in the care, improvement and learning models and engaged with health centers that are participating in the Collaboratives. A partnership between HRSA and AHRQ has implemented a multi-year evaluation strategy.

Through a partnership with CDC, the Medstar Research Institute and NIDDK, a pilot with five health centers was initiated to translate the results of the Diabetes Prevention Program into practice, utilizing the HDC strategy and models. The pilot teams have tested and implemented successful strategies to identify at risk persons, and screen them. From March through November 2003, 3167 high-risk persons have been identified, 903 (28.5%) have been screened by 2 hour 75 gram oral glucose tolerance testing, resulting in 276 (30.6%) pre-diabetes patients in the registry, and 155 (17.2%) newly diagnosed persons with diabetes. Currently, 204 (75.5%) of the patients with pre-diabetes have a self-management goal and 23 patients (8.3%) have over 150 minutes of exercise per week. Thirty-four patients (16.6%) have 7% or greater average weight loss. In the diabetes prevention pilot, the average percent weight loss goal is weight loss greater than 7%. The goal for high risks patients who develop diabetes is 1%.

AHRQ Proposals for Approach to Translation

The AHRQ Concept of the synergy and differences between phase I and phase II translation is summarized in Table 4. The heading of the left column, "Publishing Research" represents Phase I translation; the right column, "Spreading Innovation" is Phase II translation.

Table 4. From Research into Practice;
From Knowledge to System Change

Publishing Research	Spreading Innovation
Aim: Truth	Aim: Change & improvement practice
Methods: • Explanatory/predictive models • Blinded tests • No bias • All possible data • Fixed hypotheses Synergy • One large test • Stable cohort(s)	Methods: • Transformational methods • Tests Observable • Stable bias • Just enough data • Changing hypotheses • Sequential tests • Changing populations

Source: adapted from T. Nolan,
Associates In Process Improvement

We offer two proposals for improving inter-actions between the culture of basic research and the culture of quality improvement:

1. Proposal for Methods

- Involve decision makers and those with quality improvement, public health and community expertise in development of hypotheses, study design, and implementation, e.g. Canadian Health Services Research Foundation.
- Study system change and interactions in complex systems – the idea that behavior of systems is the product of the system itself, not its individual pieces.

2. Proposal for Communication, Generation and Implementation of New Ideas

- Networking, conferences, internet (quality improvement community and decision makers) as well as peer review journals (science community).
- Redesigned funding opportunities to support programs that integrate research with system change.
- The results should inform policy debates.

A high performing health center engaged in the Health Disparities Collaboratives reflected on their biggest barriers. They had to overcome the following:

- The belief that our patients cannot change and that little changes don't matter.
- The idea that we need consensus to change anything.
- The concept that improving care means more work.

- That we cannot improve without more full time staff.
- The belief in a provider-oriented rather than a patient-oriented care system.

This center overcame the barriers to system change, not in a life time, but in months. All of us at the local and national level can learn from them and be optimistic that positive change and world class results are within reach, when we are committed to a comprehensive mission driven approach.

References

1. *The Improvement Guide.* Gerald JL, Kevin MN, Thomas WN, Clifford LN, Lloyd PP. Jossey-Bass, 1996.

2. Bodenheimer T, Wagner EH, Grumback K. Improving primary care for patients with chronic illness. *JAMA* 2002, Oct 9; 288(14):1775-9.

3. Bodenheimer T, Wagner EH, Grumbach K. Improving primary care for patients with chronic illness: the chronic care model, Part 2. *JAMA* 2002 Oct 16;288(15):1909-14.

4. *http://www.healthdisparities.net*

5. *http://www.ihi.org*

Translational Research at the CDC – The Future

Frank Vinicor, MD, MPH

Director, Division of Diabetes Translation
Centers for Disease Control and Prevention

CDC Agenda for Translation

Things are getting better, but we are going to have to change if we want things to stay the same, i.e. continue to get better.

Recent studies indicate that improvements in diabetes preventive behaviors ("intermediate process indicators") are occurring in most health systems, with early suggestions of stabilization of some long-term complications ("distal outcome indicators"). Thus, the "translation glass," while not spilling over, is certainly half-full, and rising. In fact, over the history of medical translation – from preventive strategies for scurvy, to diabetic retinopathy, glycemic control in type 1 diabetes, cardiovascular disease among persons with diabetes, and now primary prevention of type 2 diabetes – the time between validated efficacy science and attention to clinical/public health practice has become progressively shorter.

To continue improvements in the rate, depth and breadth of diabetes translation, however, 3 different realities must be addressed. *First*, changes must be made in existing health systems – not only in the structure and function of these systems, but also in the very definition of a health system (which must increasingly include sites where people work, live, play and reflect). *Second*, serious commitment to prevention must occur, which involves more than "traditional" health care systems, and must be led by health practitioners as "citizen leaders." This adds a new element (citizen leader) to the previous definitions of a "health care professional" (caregiver and scientist). *Third*, regardless of more efficacious health systems for prevention and control of chronic diseases and inclusion of community elements in the very concept of a health system, continued excessive focus on individual entitlement to highly efficacious, expensive and specialty treatment (vs. reasonable levels of broad-based communitarian health) will eventually undermine progress in diabetes translation. These three issues will be the continued targets of diabetes translational public health research and programs at CDC.

From clinical trials to community:
The science of translating diabetes and obesity research

CDC Translational Targets and Underlying Basic Philosophy

The Targets

1. Us – Everyone. Change the primary role of our healthcare system to disease prevention rather than (after-the-fact) disease treatment, although the latter will always be necessary too.

2. Location – where people live, work, play and reflect.

3. The country – address the fundamental question of best to a few versus good to the many.

Basic Philosophy

"The dream of modern medicine maybe no longer viable as it stands. Even if unlimited resources were available, modern medicine cannot deliver on its most extravagant promises, nor even on many that seem modest and plausible. My contention is that modern societies need a "sustainable" medicine, a medicine that, in both research and healthcare delivery, aims for a steady-state plateau, at the level that is economically affordable and equitably available, and also at a level that is sustainable, satisfying most – but of necessity, not all - reasonable health needs and expectations."

Reference

Callahan D. False *hopes: Why america's quest for perfect health is a recipe for disaster*, Simon & Schuster, 1998, New York, NY

The Future of Translational Research at the NIDDK

Allen M. Spiegel, MD

Director
*National Institute of Diabetes
and Digestive and Kidney Diseases*

Research and Dissemination Spectrum

The spectrum of scientific activities that begins with the identification of a health problem and ends with dissemination and translation of proven interventional approaches to the problem proceeds through three sequential steps:

Step 1 – epidemiologic and basic research to identify potential risk factors, mechanisms and influence.

Step 2 – clinical trials to determine efficacy of risk factor changes on health outcomes.

Step 3 – clinical and community trials to determine effectiveness of interventional approaches to change risk factors.

NIDDK Translational Research Program

The NIDDK has for several years made funds available for translational research through the R18/R34 grant mechanism. The NIDDK's current emphasis for these R18/R34 awards is translation of the success of the Diabetes Prevention Program (DPP) in which a lifestyle intervention significantly reduced the incidence of type 2 diabetes in over 3,000 subjects at high risk for developing the disease. Investigators interested in pursuing translational research in other areas of diabetes care, such as improving glycemic control and prevention of complications in a cost-effective manner in real world settings are encouraged to apply.

The NIDDK Translational Research Program stresses the importance of developing outcome measures applicable to the community setting. Of particular importance is the need for diffusion of successful translational research – concerning outcome measures and a myriad of other translational issues – from individual community settings to the national level.

Diabetes Research and Training Centers (DRTCs), Obesity and Nutritional Research Centers (ONRCs) and Clinical Nutritional Research Units (CNRUs) funded by NIDDK provide a unique interface between Academic Health Centers where they are located and the community at large.

From clinical trials to community:
The science of translating diabetes and obesity research

NIH Obesity Research Task Force

The goals of the recently established NIH
Obesity Research Task Force are:

- Evaluate the effectiveness and assure
  translation of strategies to maintain healthy
  weight in children and adults through lifestyle
  behavior (activity, diet) change which can
  be applied in a community, home, school,
  or workplace environment.

- Use knowledge of regulation of energy
  storage and food intake to develop new therapeutic modalities (including drugs, surgery,
  and other technologies) to complement
  lifestyle interventions.

- Use knowledge of mechanisms whereby
  obesity increases risk for co-morbidities to
  develop potential therapeutic approaches for
  ameliorating these conditions independent
  of weight loss.

A website *(http://www.obesityresearch.nih.gov)*
provides information on the Task Force's
strategic plan and research information
for investigators. It will also cite links to NIH
obesity information sites for the public.

The NIH Roadmap *(http://www.nihroadmap.nih.gov)*

Raynard S. Kington, MD, PhD

Deputy Director
National Institutes of Health

Genesis of the NIH Roadmap

The fundamental need for a "roadmap" to
guide trans-NIH functions derives from the
well-documented problems (barriers) moving
scientific discovery from its origin (the bench)
to the bedside (clinical research) to the practice
community nationwide (improvement of the
nation's health). Efforts to facilitate this continuum – i.e. translational research- are not new
to the NIH. During the 1980s, the NIH, particularly the National Cancer Institute (NCI) and
the National Heart, Lung and Blood Institute
(NHLBI) proposed a sequence of translational
research activities: hypothesis generation; interventional methods development; controlled
interventional trials (RCTs); studies in defined
populations; and demonstration research.

Why a Roadmap?

The accelerated pace of discoveries in the life
sciences has prompted a need for their more
rapid translation into practice. Opportunities
now exist to build an integrated system that
is far more effective than current approaches.
The sum of our current approaches for bringing
new scientific discoveries to bear on the
nation's health are uncoordinated, inefficient,
wasteful and sometimes counterproductive.
Without a principal and comprehensive guide,
there is little reason to expect they will change.

Roadmap Chronology

August 2002
– Consultation with over 100 thought leaders.

September 2002
– Institute and Center (IC) Directors'
  Leadership Retreat Discussion.

March 2003
– Formation of 15 Working Groups
  including over 300 outside experts.

April 2003
– Presentation to Council of Public
  Representatives (COPR).

May 2003
– Working Groups propose initiatives.

June 2003
– IC Directors commit to initiatives.

June 2003
– Presentation to the Advisory Committee
  to the Director (ACD).

September 2003
– Presentation to advocacy groups/press.

FY 2004-2013
– Staged implementation.

Criteria for Roadmap Initiatives

When the Working Groups proposed Roadmap initiatives (May 2003 in the chronology above), they were asked to consider the following questions for each proposal:

- Is it "transforming" – will it change how or what biomedical research is conducted in the next decades?

- Would its outcome enhance the ability of all NIH Institutes and Centers to achieve their own missions?

- Can the NIH afford to NOT attempt it?

- Will it be compelling to our stakeholders, especially the public?

- Is it something that no other entity can or will do?

Roadmap Implementation

All Institutes and Centers committed to invest jointly in a pool of resources to support current and future Roadmap initiatives. For FY2004-FY2009 this will total $2 billion.

Many of the initiatives are **difficult** – some will fail!

Three Core Themes of the NIH Roadmap

Each core theme applies to a major component of the translation continuum.

Theme #1 – New Pathways to Technology

New building blocks and pathways; molecular libraries; bioinformatics; computational biology; nanomedicine; and several other developing technologies.

Theme # 2 – Research Teams of the Future

The scale and complexity of current science requires novel team approaches, including: interdisciplinary research teams; public-private partnerships; and programs to fund high-risk, high-impact research, such as the Director's Pioneer Award.

Interdisciplinary research teams are not altogether a new idea. Their assembly and operation require much further development. The current system of academic advancement favors the independent, not the multidisciplinary collaborative, investigator. Most institutions have scientists in discrete departments, fostering continued independence of their faculty and staff. Interdisciplinary research teams take time to assemble and require unique resources.

A new program, the NIH Director's Pioneer Award, will support individuals with untested ideas that are potentially ground breaking. It will encourage innovation and risk taking. A totally new application and peer review process will provide successful applicants $500,000/year for 5 years. Understandably, applications are expected to be highly competitive.

Theme # 3 – Re-engineering Clinical Research

The impact of this theme will be felt at both the "bedside" and "practice" components of the translational continuum. The initiative incorporates enhanced translational research centers and enabling technologies for improved attainment of clinical outcomes, such as quality of life measures discussed elsewhere in this document. Much of this will be accomplished via expansion of the function and reach of the current typical NIH Network diagrammed below.

The initiative will require linking and integrating these clinical research networks so that clinical studies and trials can be conducted more effectively. Such linkage will ensure that patients, physicians and scientists form true "Communities of Research." Translational research topics will have an established infrastructure with strong community linkages from which they can be pursued.

These Integrated Clinical Research Networks can be used to rapidly address questions beyond their traditional scope. The interoperable "Network of Networks," diagrammed below, can share sites, develop common data standards and informatics, and prepare software application tools for protocol preparation, IRB management and adverse event reporting.

A reinvigorated clinical research enterprise will require a diverse group of trained and certified community health care providers across the country who will enroll and follow their own patients in clinical trials and accelerate translation of results into their practice.

Multidisciplinary teams are required for clinical research.

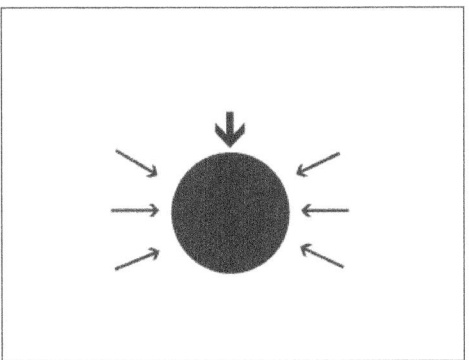

The Trans-NIH Multidisciplinary K12 Career Development Program will support training of investigators from a variety of disciplines – MD, PhD, RN, MPH, DC, etc. – to function in multidisciplinary team settings. The NIH Program features up to 5 years of training; core didactic courses and project-specific training; mentored research experience in team settings; faculty and mentor support to protect their time; tuition support; annual meetings; and the opportunity to engage in translational studies.

The goal of harmonization of the clinical research regulatory process will be achieved through simplification of requirements for clinical research in ways that enhance public trust. Coordination and clarification of numerous elements of the regulatory process are involved, such as adverse event reporting; human subjects protection (DSMB-IRB interactions, consent procedures); auditing and monitoring clinical trials; HIPAA, privacy and conflict of interest policies; investigator registration and financial disclosure; and standards for electronic data submission and reporting.

Summary

Building vibrant communities of clinical research requires participation, consultation, collaboration, and funding from patients, health care providers, foundations, industry, academia, and federal partners – *all stakeholders*. A key goal of the NIH Roadmap is to foster these dynamic interactions to strengthen all types of clinical research and to create the infrastructure of national networks to support their research including translational research.

Key Points from Panel Discussions

Editor's note

During the one and one-half day conference, four interactive conference attendees/speaker-panel sessions occurred. These sessions followed sequential sections of the conference agenda and had the titles listed below. Names in parentheses indicate the speakers who presented during the section being discussed.

1. Fundamental Issues in Translational Research
   (Roland G. Hiss and Lawrence W. Green)

2. Outcomes for Translational Research
   (Russell E. Glasgow, K.M. Venkat Narayan, and David Meltzer)

3. Experimental Design Issues
   in Translational Research
   (Marshall Chin and Carol Mangione)

4. Review and Critique of Translational
   Research Studies
   (Barbara K. Rimer, Alan Delamater, and Harold C. Sox)

Each of these four sessions resulted in active audience and speaker exchange involving questions and comments on aspects of the presentations, ideas for further research (arising from both the audience and the speakers), identification of cross-cutting issues and reactions from the NIDDK administrators and other NIH officials. A collegial and inspired exchange ensued.

Points made, questions asked, and responses offered did not fall neatly under the content headings listed above. Frequent reference back and forth to points discussed in prior panel sessions occurred throughout, an outcome that the conference organizers both predicted and sought. Consequently, the often fragmentary points made have been combined into a reasonable content organization under the following five headings:

1. NIDDK program announcement concerning translational research.

2. Efficacy/effectiveness continuum.

3. Community-based effectiveness trials.

4. Best practices.

5. Sustainability of interventions.

The guiding rationale for choosing the organizational headings just listed and placement of individual points within them included:

1. What will the readers of this document acquire that they can incorporate into their own thinking and planning?

2. What statements received substantial endorsement from the conference attendees?

No attempt was made to be archival, nor to attribute any point to individual speakers or audience participants. The interactive dynamics of the conference fostered a shared sense of group effort towards common goals. In addition, the design and conduct of the conference did not seek a "research agenda for the future" although many suggestions in that regard arose from the conference discussions.

Key Point 1
Translational Research Program Announcement

The NIDDK has stimulated translational research (Phase II type) through its program announcements entitled "Translational Research for the Prevention and Control of Diabetes", PA-02-053 and "Planning Grants for Translational Research for the Prevention and Control of Diabetes", PA-03-052. The program announcements utilize the R18 and R34 funding mechanism. The desire to assist investigators considering a response to these program announcements determined much of the agenda for this conference.

Key Point 2
Efficacy/Effectiveness Continuum

Efficacy and effectiveness studies, as defined in the chapter of that name authored by Dr. Lawrence W. Green, are not dichotomous. There is no "firewall" between them. Efficacy studies begin the translational process with research performed under controlled conditions with emphasis on internal validity. They greatly influence the content of effectiveness studies, conducted largely in the community setting, and frequently blend with those studies resulting in field trials that have both efficacy and effectiveness components. The randomized controlled trial (RCT) methodology dominates the research design for well-executed efficacy studies; strict adherence to the RCT-design for effectiveness studies, however, can create an artificial situation that is no longer representative of the same trial conducted in other settings. Inordinate utilization of efficacy trial methodology in effectiveness trials creates a requirement for control over experimental conditions that is not possible or may limit the utility or external validity in community-based effectiveness trials. Although the inappropriate use of the RCT-design in effectiveness trials is generally recognized, effectiveness trials not employing an RCT face considerable reviewer bias during the consideration of competitive grant applications to NIH (and often other major national funding agencies).

Properly designed and executed effectiveness studies at the community level require consideration of a myriad of community-derived factors. Large sample sizes, multiple sites, nonhomogeneous populations, cultural, financial and socioeconomic diversity are some of the complicating factors involved. Conference attendees, both speakers and audience participants, recommended additional inclusions in a competitive comprehensive grant application for a community-based effectiveness study: cost analysis of the intervention; studies emphasizing issues within special populations; and dissemination plans following a successful trial. These multiple considerations create a conflict between a large, expensive, long and multi-faceted effectiveness trial and the availability of funding of such an endeavor – and word-length limitations of any subsequent manuscript.

The tension between reviewer bias, or reviewer inexperience, concerning research design of effectiveness trials and the availability of adequate funding to conduct them was extensively described at this conference, but not resolved.

Key Point 3
Community-Based Effectiveness Trials

Identification of the problem to be addressed and development of the intervention(s) to address the problem should be a joint enterprise between the academically-oriented researcher and the community – joint development of the application for funding and joint execution of the real world effectiveness trial. The "community-centered" characteristic of the researcher/community "team" parallels the "patient-centered" characteristic of a clinical "team." Both are interdependent partnerships. Development of the researcher/community partnership requires blending of the objectives of the two partners – research with publishable results versus tangible improvement of community healthcare. Meaningful partnerships also require hard work and time to develop.

To enhance community preparedness to participate in an equal partnership with academic colleagues, conference attendees offered these proposals:

1. Development of a community infrastructure to support community-based effectiveness trials, similar in concept to general clinical research centers (GCRCs) support of clinical research. In that way, each effectiveness trial would not have to develop its own community partner.

2. Development of research skills for community-based partners. This includes technical assistance, statistical support, grant writing workshops (that many professional societies offer on a regular basis) and, most importantly, critical feedback to community-based applicants about correctable weaknesses in their proposal and to the academic applicants to enhance their understanding of community health care issues. (Incidental note on the latter point: principal investigators applying for major funding must have a publication record that documents their qualifications to conduct the study being proposed.)

Several national organizations supporting the academic/community-based partnerships described at the conference included:

1. National Practice-Based Research Networks (PBRNs)

2. Agency for Healthcare Research and Quality (AHRQ, which also funds the PBRNs)

3. Robert Wood Johnson Foundation

Best Practices

Best practices are derived from multiple sources – the Cochrane Reviews, the Canadian Taskforce on the Periodic Health Exam, the U.S. Preventative Services Taskforce, the Guide to Community Preventive Services, and clinical guideline development by a host of national, regional and local professional organizations. A growing professional ethic stipulates that "best practices" should be "evidenced-based." Considerable controversy surrounds both terms. One aspect of the controversy relates to the definition of what is a best practice. Best practice for whom? Under what conditions? And the validity of the best practice from the perspective of the community-based healthcare provider. Another element of the controversy relates to the means by which these practices will be "translated," i.e. adopted, by the practice community.

Traditional continuing medical education in all its forms constitutes a first step in the widespread adoption process, but is unable to complete that process. Responsibility for failure to adopt validated best practices has been placed, rather indiscriminately, on a variety of healthcare agencies and individual practitioners. However, such misplaced blame does not solve the problem, rather it fosters a confrontational atmosphere. Conference attendees agreed that improvement in the overall U.S. healthcare delivery system – adoption of "best practices," integration of healthcare services, cost-effective practices, and attention to a myriad of other changes – is a systems problem, not an individual problem.

Sustainability of Interventions

The issue of sustainability of community-based interventions to improve healthcare at the community level permeated much of the discussions of the key points described above. An efficacy study can have a beginning and an end, and usually does. A community-based effectiveness trial, however, should include a demonstration of how the intervention(s) may be maintained after the formal study has been completed. Conference discussion of this issue can be organized under two headings: 1) creation of a community-based infrastructure left behind upon formal study completion; and 2) perspective of the recipient of the benefit of sustained intervention – the individual patient or the funding agency.

1. Community Infrastructure Left Behind

From a societal perspective, the best final outcome of a successful community-based effectiveness trial is ownership of the program by the community and the means (money and infrastructure) to sustain it. If such an outcome is not achieved, the transferability of the results of this study to other communities is diminished. Lack of the means to sustain successful interventions damages the interest other communities might have in replicating the original study. (Mounting an all-out effort for a one-time benefit is not appealing.) Thus, sustainability of interventions becomes another inclusion requirement for effectiveness trial funding proposals. The Robert Wood Johnson Foundation has adopted this criteria during review of community-based proposals that it may sup-

port. (Incidental note was made during these discussions of how thin the "sustainability literature" was.)

2. Perspective of Benefit Recipient

Benefit of a sustained intervention varies considerably depending upon who/what is to receive this benefit – and particularly when this benefit will be realized. An individual patient will probably sustain the intervention applicable to him/her if they receive benefit from it now or in the immediate future; however if the benefit will not be realized until the distant future, interest in the intervention will probably fade. From the perspective of a healthcare funding agency (such as an HMO) similar time considerations apply. A healthcare financing agency will show great interest in an intervention that reduces their current costs, but much less interest in an intervention that may reduce their distant future costs. As a consequence of these understandable attitudes by both individual patients and healthcare funding agencies, sustaining interventions with distant benefit is extremely hard to do. And the means to do so currently does not exist.

Conference Planners and Faculty

Marshall H. Chin, MD, MPH ◉ ◆
Department of Medicine
Chicago Diabetes Research
and Training Center
University of Chicago
5841 South Maryland Avenue
MC2007, Room B216
Chicago, IL 60637
T 773.702.4769
F 773.834.2238
mchin@medicine.bsd.uchicago.edu

Alan M. Delamater, PhD ◆
Department of Pediatrics
Division of Clinical Psychology
University of Miami School of Medicine
Post Office Box 016820
Miami, FL 33101
T 305.243.6857
F 305.243.4512
adelamater@med.miami.edu

Barbara J. DeVinney, PhD ◉
Office of Behavioral and
Social Sciences Research
National Institutes of Health
1267 Snapdragon Lane
Christiansburg, VA 24073
T 540.731.3109
DevinneB@od.nih.gov

Lawrence J. Fine, MD, DrPH ◉
Office of Behavioral and
Social Sciences Research
Office of the Director
National Institutes of Health

Current Address:
Clinical Applications and Prevention Program
National Heart, Lung and Blood Institute
National Institutes of Health
6701 Rockledge Drive
2 Rockledge Center, Room 8138
Bethesda, MD 20892
T 301.435.0305
F 301.480.1669
finel@nhlbi.nih.gov

Sanford A. Garfield, PhD ◉ ▣
Division of Diabetes, Endocrinology,
and Metabolic Diseases
National Institute of Diabetes
and Digestive and Kidney Diseases
National Institutes of Health
2 Democracy Plaza
6707 Democracy Boulevard, Room 685
Bethesda, MD 20892-5460
T 301.594.8803
F 301.402.6271
garfields@extra.niddk.nih.gov

Russell E. Glasgow, PhD ⬤ ◆
Clinical Research Unit
Kaiser Permanente Colorado
335 Road Runner Lane
Penrose, CO 81240
T 719.372.3165
F 719.372.6395
russg@ris.net

Lawrence W. Green, DrPH ⬤ ▲ ◆
Public Health Practice Program Office
Centers for Disease Control and Prevention

Current Address:
Visiting Professor
School of Public Health
University of California at Berkeley
66 Santa Paula Avenue
San Francisco, CA 94127
T 415.566.6178
F 415.566.6178
LWGreen@comcast.net

Roland G. Hiss, MD ⬤ ▲ ◆
Department of Medical Education
University of Michigan Medical School
Towsley Center, Box 0201
Ann Arbor, MI 48109
T 734.769.0570
F 734.936.1641
redhiss@umich.edu

Raynard S. Kington, MD, PhD ◆
Deputy Director
National Institues of Health
Department of Health and Human Services
1 Center Drive
Building One, Room 126
Bethesda, MD 20892-0148
T 301.496.7322
F 301.402.2700
kingtonr@mail.nih.gov

Robert Kuczmarski, DrPH ⬤
Division of Digestive Diseases and Nutrition
National Institute of Diabetes
and Digestive and Kidney Diseases
National Institues of Health
6707 Democracy Boulevard
Room 673, MSC 5450
Bethesda, MD 20892-5450
T 301.451.8354
F 301.480.8300
rk191r@nih.gov

Saul Malozowski, MD, PhD, MBA ⬤ ▨
National Institute of Diabetes
and Digestive and Kidney Diseases
National Institutes of Health
2 Democracy Plaza
6707 Democracy Boulevard
Room 679, MSC 5450
Bethesda, MD 20892
T 301.451.4683
F 301.480.3503
malozowski@extra.niddk.nih.gov

From clinical trials to community:
The science of translating diabetes and obesity research

- – Conference Planning Committee
- – Conference Conveners
- – Conference Co-Director
- – Conference Faculty

Carol M. Mangione, MD, MSPH
Department of Medicine
Resource Center for Minority Aging Research
David Geffin School of Medicine at the
University of California Los Angeles
911 Broxton Avenue
Los Angeles, CA 90024
T 310.794.2298
F 310.794.0723
cmangione@mednet.ucla.edu

David G. Marrero, PhD
Department of Medicine
Division of Endocrinology
Indiana Diabetes Prevention
and Control Center
Indiana University School of Medicine
250 University Boulevard, Room 122
Indianapolis, IN 46202
T 317.278.0900
F 317.278.0911
dgmarrer@iupui.edu

David Meltzer, MD, PhD
Department of Medicine
School of Public Policy
and Department of Economics
University of Chicago
5841 South Maryland Avenue, MC 2007
Chicago, IL 60637
T 773.702.0836
F 773.834.2238
dmeltzer@medicine.bsd.uchicago.edu

K. M. Venkat Narayan, MD, MPH, MBA
Division of Diabetes Translation
Centers for Disease Control and Prevention
2858 Woodcock Boulevard
Mail Stop K-10
Atlanta, GA 30341
T 770.488.1051
F 770.488.1148
kav4@cdc.gov

Judith M. Ottoson, EdD, MPH
Institute for Public Health
Georgia State University

Current Address:
66 Santa Paula Avenue
San Francisco, CA 94127
T 415.566.6178
F 415.566.6178
padjmo@langate.gsu.edu

Ken Resnicow, PhD
Department of Health Behavior
and Health Education
University of Michigan School of Public Health
1420 Washington Heights (SPH II), Room 5009
Ann Arbor, MI 48109-2029
T 734.647.0212
F 734.763.7379
kresnic@umich.edu

From clinical trials to community:
The science of translating diabetes and obesity research

Barbara K. Rimer, DrPH ◆
School of Public Health; Lineberger
Comprehensive Cancer Center
The University of North Carolina at Chapel Hill
CB #7295, 102 Mason Farm Road
Chapel Hill, NC 27599-7295
T 919.843.8088
F 919.966.4244
brimer@unc.edu

Harold C. Sox, MD, MACP ◆
American College of Physicians
190 North Independence Mall West
Philadelphia, PA 19106-1572
T 215.351.2620
F 215.351.2644
hsox@acponline.org

Allen M. Spiegel, MD ◆
Director
National Institute of Diabetes
and Digestive and Kidney Diseases
National Institutes of Health
Building 31, Room 9A52
31 Center Drive, MSC 2560
Bethesda, MD 20892-2560
T 301.496.5877
F 301.402.2125
spiegela@extra.niddk.nih.gov

David M. Stevens, MD, MA ◆
Center for Quality Improvement
and Patient Safety
Agency for Healthcare
Research and Quality
540 Gaither Road
Rockville, MD 20850
T 301.427.1300
F 301.427.1341
dstevens@ahrq.gov

Frank Vinicor, MD, MPH ◆
Centers for Disease Control and Prevention
Division of Diabetes Translation
4770 Buford Highway, NW
Mail Stop K-10
Atlanta, GA 30341
T 770.488.5000
F 770.488.5966
fxv1@cdc.gov